PRESCHOOL LANGUAGE DISORDERS
RESOURCE GUIDE

Specific Language Impairment

SINGULAR RESOURCE GUIDE SERIES

EDITOR

Ken M. Bleile, Ph.D.
Department of Communicative Disorders
University of Northern Iowa
Cedar Falls, Iowa

ASSOCIATE EDITORS

Brian Goldstein, Ph.D.
Communication Sciences
Temple University
Philadelphia, Pennsylvania

Sharon Glennen, Ph.D.
Department of Communication Sciences
and Disorders
Towson University
Towson, Maryland

Carole Roth, Ph.D.
Department of Speech Pathology
Hennepin County Medical Center
Minneapolis, Minnesota

Amy Weiss, Ph.D.
Department of Speech Pathology and Audiology
University of Iowa
Iowa City, Iowa

Tricia Zebrowski, Ph.D.
Department of Speech Pathology and Audiology
University of Iowa
Iowa City, Iowa

Preschool Language Disorders Resource Guide

Specific Language Impairment

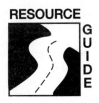

RESOURCE GUIDE

Amy L. Weiss, Ph.D., CCC-SLP

Associate Professor
Department of Speech Pathology and Audiology
The University of Iowa
Iowa City, Iowa 52242

SINGULAR

THOMSON LEARNING

Australia Canada Mexico Singapore Spain United Kingdom United States

SINGULAR

THOMSON LEARNING

Preschool Language Disorders Resource Guide: Specific Language Impairment
by Amy Weiss, Ph.D.

Business Unit Director:
William Brottmiller

Executive Marketing Manager:
Dawn Gerrain

Production Manager:
Barbara Bullock

Acquisitions Editor:
Marie Linvill

Channel Manager:
Tara Carter

Production Editor:
Sandy Doyle

Editorial Assistant:
Kristin Banach

COPYRIGHT © 2001 by Singular, an imprint of Delmar, a division of Thomson Learning, Inc. Thomson Learning™ is a trademark used herein under license

Printed in Canada
 2 3 4 5 XXX 05 04 03 02 01

For more information contact Singular,
401 West "A" Street, Suite 325
San Diego, CA 92101-7904
Or find us on the World Wide Web
at http://www.singpub.com

ALL RIGHTS RESERVED. No part of this work covered by the copyright here-on may be reproduced or used in any form or by any means—graphic, electronic, or mechanical, including photocopying, recording, taping, Web distribution or information storage and retrieval systems—without written permission of the publisher.

For permission to use material from this text or product, contact us by
Tel (800) 730-2214
Fax (800) 730-2215
www.thomsonrights.com

Library of Congress
Cataloging-in-Publication Data
Weiss, Amy L.
Preschool language disorder resource guide : specific language impairment / Amy L. Weiss.
p. cm.
Includes bibliographical references and index.
ISBN 0-7693-0029-4 (alk. paper)
1. Specific language impairment in children. 2. Preschool children—Language. I. Title.
RJ506.S68 W44 2000
618.92'855—dc21
00-059505

NOTICE TO THE READER

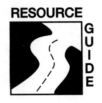

CONTENTS

SECTION 3: CASE STUDIES   143

SECTION 4: FORMS FOR EVALUATING PRESCHOOLERS' LANGUAGE AND THEIR SUCCESS IN TREATMENT   149

SECTION 5: GLOSSARY   157

SECTION 6: INTERNET RESOURCES   161

REFERENCES   165

INDEX   173

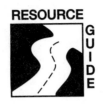

FOREWORD

The emblem for this series is a stylized road ending in an arrow. This symbol is intended to represent the goal of the series: to create books that serve as road maps to the care of communicative disorders. Like good road maps, each book gives the clinician an honest depiction of the territory, shows the various routes, and allows you the traveler to select the route best suited for your particular type of journey. Each book author is someone who knows the territory about which he or she is writing, both as a clinician and a researcher. The editorial board that advises the editors and authors is composed of some of the most respected persons in our profession. The hope of all involved in the series is that you will find the books useful and readable. Good traveling!

Ken M. Bleile, Ph.D.
Series Editor

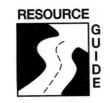

RESOURCE GUIDE

A VIGNETTE FOR PONDERING THE WONDER OF EARLY LANGUAGE LEARNING

Context: Melanie and Amy are having breakfast; Amy is across the table from her, but she is engrossed in reading the Sunday *New York Times* and not paying much attention to her niece.

Melanie (age 2 years 11 months, tries to get her aunt's attention): Aunt Amy, it *seems* like I don't have any more cheese on my plate.

Amy (dropping the paper down to take a look at Melanie and her plate): Melanie, do you want some more cheese?

Melanie: Yes.

Amy: Well, then why don't you ask for some and not say "It *seems* like I don't have any more cheese?"

Melanie: Because that's the way I ask.

The moral of the story is that young, preschool-age children learn at a very early age the fine art of using indirect requests as a type of politeness, perhaps to avoid the confrontation (and possible lack of compliance) that direct requesting can bring. In this instance Melanie has taken an indirect approach and is a little precocious in her use of hinting. Note the metalinguistic awareness evident in her response to her aunt's question. At not quite 3 years of age, Melanie recognized that she can use language to ask for things and that there are different ways to do that.

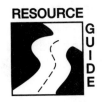

RESOURCE
GUIDE

PREFACE

WHY PRESCHOOL LANGUAGE DISORDERS?

You have already read in the foreword to this resource guide written by Ken Bleile, Series Editor, a little bit about the history of this series and our rationale in putting it together. In this particular guide we focus on the child, ages 3 through 5, who is at risk for, suspected of, or already diagnosed with a language disorder.

This is a fascinating age, an age when a lot of language learning is supposed to be taking place and the child is beginning to come into his or her own personhood. Big changes are happening in terms of the child's cognitive, social-emotional, and motor development in addition to the learning of language. It is exciting to watch the young child participate in language-based activities with family, friends, and for many this participation extends to interactions with preschool and day care classmates, teachers, and aides. In fact, after over 20 years of working with this population myself as well as training others to do likewise, I have developed a profound respect for the overwhelming majority of young children who apparently have no difficulty with the language-learning task. For me it is almost less of a mystery that there is a population of children that *does* have a difficult time learning language. The task of learning to become a competent language user is so complex that it is the fact that so many children seem to pass through its rigors unscathed that is the true mystery to me, not that a relatively small proportion of children have difficulty with the process.

The fact that the majority of children learn language normally does not make the presence of a language disorder any less serious. When a language disorder is present in young children, many are then vulnerable for a number of concomitant developmental problems. Children who have difficulty learning language are also at risk for problems in developing friendships, for example, as well as other milestones of social-emotional development. Reading and writing may also be delayed.

What we know about normal child language development and how we characterize the nature of language disorders have become areas of burgeoning research. Further, there has been increased interest in treatment efficacy research over the last 10 to 15 years and many of the investigators responsible for this new information have focused on working with the preschool-age child. That is, we not only want to know what treatment works, but also what works most effectively and efficiently for each of our young clients. Researchers have recognized that individual learning styles undoubtedly play a role in treatment efficacy and thus single subject designs have become a more accepted, mainstreamed approach to efficacy research.

You know that the intended audience for this guide as well as the rest of the series is not the undergraduate or graduate student-in-training, but instead the practicing clinician who already has had some clinical experience under her or his belt. That is why you will find this guide written so that a number of assumptions have been made about the reader's background knowledge, especially where the basics of clinical diagnosis and intervention are concerned. So, for example, when issues of best practices for generalization are enumerated in a later section, there will be no attempt to explain response or stimulus generalization. It will be assumed that the reader understands these concepts that are common to treatment approaches regardless of communication disorder area. We assume, too, that most of our readers will be speech-language pathologists and so the abbreviation of "SLP" has been used throughout.

My job has been to compile what I believe is a summary of the basic information needed by clinicians who may have never had much professional clinical experience with the preschool-age child and in particular with the child diagnosed as Specifically Language Impaired or SLI, but who now find themselves needing an update to cope with changes in their caseload or for persons who have been away from this clinical population for a while. Still other clinicians may be looking for an opportunity to keep current with this population whether or not they are experiencing an immediate need for the material. Regardless of which category may fit you, when you peruse this resource guide, it is my hope that you will come away with some useful information that could be immediately applicable to your clinical caseload where preschool-age children with language disorders are concerned.

HOW TO GET THE MOST FROM THIS GUIDE

This resource guide has been divided into four main sections, with the first, "Core Knowledge," covering basic definitions and descriptions of the disorder, then a section of assessment and intervention procedural suggestions, a glossary of terms (*Note:* Terms contained in the glossary are boldfaced in the text), and finally sections containing both additional resource listings via the Internet and blank forms that can be copied and used for language data analysis or for charting behaviors during treatment. As much as possible, care has been taken to refer the reader to other helpful portions within this guide as well as to references available in other published forms and sources. You will notice that a number of Web site addresses and descriptions of those sites have been included in the appendix where those sites contain useful information for persons working with children who have preschool language disorders. Again, the reader will notice that some particular attention has been paid to those children diagnosed as Specifically Language Impaired, hereafter referred to exclusively as SLI.

One of the other format features you will notice in this resource guide is that the initial section, "Core Knowledge," will read most like a traditional text. However, once you read beyond this section and enter into the assessment and intervention portions of the guide, you will notice a change in the format and the information provided will be in an abbreviated manner—short and to the point, most in bulleted format, with clinical insights and examples given afterwards to explicate the "here's how to" portions. Here, too, additional references will be provided to help the reader "flesh out" those topics where individuals may desire more information. As much as possible throughout the guide, references to validate the statements made and suggestions given will also be provided to assist clinicians in their evaluation of the practices described as they pick and choose among available procedures. We hope you will find this approach useful in your work.

Amy L. Weiss, Ph.D., CCC-SLP

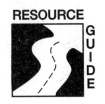

RESOURCE
GUIDE

ACKNOWLEDGMENTS

I would like to convey my deepest appreciation to my colleague and fellow Iowan, Ken Bleile, for considering me an appropriate "brainstormer" for this series as well as an associate editor and author for one of the resource guides. On some days it has been his faith in my ability that has gotten me through some of the more challenging publishing rough spots.

My colleagues, friends, family, and mostly my students at the University of Iowa have shown infinite patience when I've had to underextend myself over the past year or more to get this writing project completed.

Most of all I would like to thank the people in my life who have been most responsible for facilitating my love for the preschool population: Beth Gage and Nancy Green, now far removed (in North Carolina and Colorado, respectively) from the Colonel Wolfe School in Champaign, Illinois, where they both supervised and befriended me in the mid-1970s when I was a Master of Arts student at the University of Illinois; Joan Good Erickson, my professor, advisor, and chief cheering section during my two years at the University of Illinois and beyond; and Larry Leonard, my always generous doctoral mentor at Purdue University whose dedication to figuring out the whys and hows of language disorders, especially SLI, continues to be an inspiration to me. I would be remiss not to give my mother, Mrs. Barbara Weiss, a special thank you because she undoubtedly is the person who instilled in me early on my great love for listening to young children's language and trying to figure out what they are *really* trying to say. Hopefully, this volume will be a credit to all they have taught me.

**To Melanie Anne, Jeremy Brian,
and
Joseph William**

*. . . who, without knowing it, taught me and many of my
students over the years to appreciate the mystery and wonder
of language learning by their examples—many examples.
I officially thank you.*

SECTION

CORE KNOWLEDGE

∙∙

This first section of the book includes some of the basic information needed by clinicians who are facing the challenge of the assessment, evaluation, and treatment of children who are preschool aged and language disordered. Information about normal language development is provided as is information concerning current definitions of language disorders, current controversies involving theories about why there are language disorders, and especially why there is so much interest in the phenomenon of specific language impairment or SLI.

FIRST THINGS FIRST:
A FEW WORDS ABOUT NORMAL LANGUAGE DEVELOPMENT

No one who plans to work with the preschool-age child with a language disorder can do so without reference to what normally developing children are able to do with language at this stage in their development. So, if you feel the need for an update in preschool language disorders because you just have not spent much time around preschool children, you need to also consider spending some extended quality time with preschool-age children who are developing language normally.

My specific recommendation would be to observe these youngsters in a variety of settings, for example, in their homes, in day care classrooms, or out of doors at play, where the demands on their communication competencies are bound to differ and a diverse set of competencies may be revealed. Note their general ability to express themselves with finesse, perhaps explaining what they want or need, have or feel, and how they view the world around them, by relying on a sizable vocabulary (sometimes surprisingly so), a variety of sentence types and constructions, and a number of conversation strategies.

Likewise, the demands on young children's comprehension skills will vary from setting to setting and although you may need to pay even more careful attention, especially to the surrounding context, your observations should help increase your appreciation for both the extent and limitations of young children's comprehension abilities. You know, as all SLPs with any experience in the area of comprehension do, that comprehension is a much more subtle competency to evaluate than are production abilities. As Chapman (1978) first pointed out, young children's attempts to comprehend in the absence of full linguistic knowledge often leads to their use of comprehension strategies that take into account what they do know and help them speculate on the rest. Use of comprehension strategies may aid the child in appearing to know much more than what he or she actually comprehends based on linguistic information alone. Sometimes what the child knows is nonlinguistic and context based so the child who waves "bye-bye" when father holds him and verbally encourages him to perform this gesture while he himself models the action is probably responding imitatively to the father's model and not to the verbal command to "wave bye-bye." However, the caregiver, eager to see the child perform, will often interpret the scene as proof of linguistic comprehension.

The use of these comprehension strategies is one of the child's ways of **bootstrapping** from what is known into the more challenging unknown. Sometimes the strategy works well, and the child appears to figure out the language puzzle. At other times the outcome tips the child's hand, that is, it makes clear that true language knowledge is not at the sophisticated level that had been assumed. What the use of the strategy does provide for the child, however, is a method for testing the child's current hypothesis of what is a correct contribution to the interaction. And, we assume that these hypotheses will be adjusted according to the explicit or implicit feedback that may be provided. This contribution also is just that—a way to take a turn in an ongoing conversation when one's repertoire for contributions is incomplete.

I have also found it very useful, in addition to spending more time observing the children themselves, to spend some time learning more about the input preschoolers are exposed to on television, in movies and videos, and through popular children's literature. This sort of information has been invaluable to me in my attempts to decipher preschoolers' stories, which for many young children are rambling, immature collections of facts [Applebee (1978) called these "heaps"] with little of the predicted narrative structure we expect to see in older, more sophisticated children's stories. However, do not be too surprised when normally developing children later in the preschool age range are producing fully formed episodic structures and examples of mature narratives (Westby, 1994), showing budding knowledge of a **story grammar**.

One of the dangers of infrequent work with the preschool-age population is that it is relatively easy to forget the incredible amount of language knowledge displayed by a normally developing child within this age range (roughly 3 to 5 years old) and thus underestimate the level of performance that should be expected when you are working with a clinical case where the diagnosis has been a language disorder. As with any disorder area, the more experience you accrue with the population, the better you will be able to validly evaluate performance and progress. Once you have a prerequisite amount of clinical experience behind you, and you have reached a clinical "comfort zone" with this population, clinical judgment skills become a reliable adjunct to standardized testing (Records & Weiss, 1990). That is to say, you will develop a set of internalized expectations for how children in the preschool years should behave in a typical communication venue. This process of developing insight is the same for child language disorders as it is for any disorder area when we add to our experience base.

There are several guiding principles to remember when we consider language development. First, when we talk about **language** we are talking about a systematically derived code for communication, where symbols—written, spoken, or signed—are used in a socially conventional way. The latter is what enables us to communicate: language communities agree on the meanings of the symbols they use and the rules for their combinations. Thus, the problem with the idiolects sometimes developed by the rare set of twins ("twin language") or children in other multiple birth groups would be that, although their system may be rule governed and certainly creative, it is not shared with others outside of the twin pair and so has limited communicative utility.

Remember, too, that languages are dynamic systems, undergoing changes over time in any one or all of their component subsystems that lend organization to sentence construction or the sounds used in the language, or the vocabulary used. For example, we rarely hear the word "shall" used except in the most formal of situations although it was common at the beginning of the twentieth century. In recent years there has been a steady infiltration of words into the English language thanks to the computer culture and space exploration. "Hacker," the specialized hardware meaning of "interface," and the term "lunar module" are examples that come to mind. It might be a good idea to add here that vocabulary development is one of those language areas that has the potential to continue enhancement over the course of the life span. Of course, the trick as we age becomes being able to retrieve the steadily increasing vocabulary we have amassed at will!

To provide the most appropriate services to all of our clients, and especially to those learning language, the issue of *language difference* versus *language disorder* is one that should be thoroughly understood by the speech-language clinician (ASHA Position Paper on Dialects, 1983). We each use a dialect of our language; designation of standard versus nonstandard dialects bears no relationship to the inherent value of one dialect of a language over another. In almost all cases, nonstandard dialects are far more like the standard than they are different from it. Unfortunately, myths about social valuation of standard dialects and devaluation of nonstandard dialects persist (see Wolfram, 1991) and can result in inaccurate diagnoses, treatment provision, or denial of treatment (see Vaughn-Cooke, 1986).

Clinical Insight

The misguided notion of there being an inherent linguistic value of the standard dialect was highlighted during the media's focus on the Ebonics controversy in Oakland, California, in the late 1990s. Ebonics is a term used to describe what other researchers and linguists refer to as Black English (BE), Black English Vernacular (BEV), or African-American English (AAE), a nonstandard dialect of English, very frequently but not always spoken by persons who consider themselves to be African-Americans. When the school board for Oakland, California, suggested that Ebonics be used as a tool to help those children who already used this nonstandard dialect for learning Standard English (SE) and especially for the purpose of gaining better access to literacy learning, the resulting uproar, in my opinion largely relating to the media's ignorance of the topic of dialects, languages, and bidialectalism and bilingualism, misrepresented the intent of the school

(continued)

(continued)

board's proposal. The opposition proclaimed that the children of Oakland who were being encouraged to use Ebonics, their "home language," would never learn SE as a result and were therefore doomed to stagnate (sic) in an educational sense in the short term and in an economic sense in the long term. The fact remains that the mainstream SE-speaking society in the United States generally devalues the use of Ebonics. Historically, persons who exclusively speak this dialect of English in mainstream contexts can still expect fewer opportunities for getting ahead in a national workplace dominated by SE-speaking expectations. In fact, what the school board of Oakland was suggesting by their proposal was the use of **contrastive analysis** to teach children who were already speaking Ebonics how to code switch into SE when the circumstances called for such a switch as well as to be able to recognize equivalent forms between the two dialects to enhance literacy learning. Note that this in and of itself is not a revolutionary approach. Other school districts have been using this methodology and perspective for years. The key is to view Ebonics for what it is: a bona fide language system worthy of the same respect as any other language system, as are its speakers.

What is important for the speech-language clinician to remember is that *language differences are not language disorders.* That is, the presence of the features of a systematically derived, generative, rule-governed, conventional, nonstandard dialect does not constitute a language problem, language deficit, impairment, or language disorder but instead represents a grammatical, if sometimes different way from the standard, of expressing oneself within one's community. This issue impacts the assessment, evaluation, and treatment of all of our clients and is addressed more specifically in another member of the resource guide series (see Goldstein, 2000).

THE RELATIONSHIP BETWEEN LANGUAGE DEVELOPMENT AND OTHER AREAS OF PRESCHOOL DEVELOPMENT

We must also remember that language development is inextricably tied together with cognitive development, social-emotional development, and aspects of motor development. Thus, a language disorder may be part of an all-around or pervasive disorder of development (and PDD is another classification to be tackled in a separate resource guide). SLI, however, is largely believed to be different: a language problem in the absence of other developmental or sensory concerns.

Although you may not be qualified or permitted in your work setting to directly evaluate cognitive functioning, you can gain some information about the child's general cognitive functioning by observing symbolic play and other play behaviors. As children's play routines become more complex, involving more steps for completion of a scenario or involving more protagonists and actions, we assume that their underlying language formulation skills are also somewhat more complex. So, we look for evidence of these scenarios; for example, when we observe a child feeding a baby doll and putting it to sleep, we note whether the child is playing appropriately with a variety of toys, demonstrating appropriate use of objects (such as, what actions are associated with which objects?), playing cooperatively or in parallel with other children, and so on. This is a notion that is closely tied to a conceptualization of the close relationship between certain cognitive attainments and language development. See Roth and Clark (1987) for a review of protocols for comparisons of the play behaviors found in groups of children identified as language impaired or developing language normally.

Another important factor to keep in mind is that, while we know that the language of the preschool-age child is generally developing rapidly (consider how much has to be learned in so short of a time frame!), we also know that children show evidence of individual differences in these rapidly developing patterns. That is, there is a great deal of variability in the acquisition rates that young children display as well as in the quality of the language they produce or comprehend at young ages. This is why the milestones that we so often cite, such as producing the first true word at 12 months of age or combining words at 18 months, are really averages of performance with normal ranges of performance falling on either side of the norm. This variability is evident in motor skill and other areas of development as well. It will be important, of course, to keep in mind that children who are delayed beyond the norm bear some watching. The argument for individual differences is an important one but not meant to exclude children from intervention who are presenting with early signs of developmental delay. This argument will be repeated in the following section that focuses on the "**late talker**."

Especially where the milestone concerning the advent of **real word use** is concerned, SLPs should probably focus as much attention on the presence or absence of infants' and toddlers' attempts to intentionally communicate rather than be exclusively concerned with whether the child is producing words when the first birthday is reached. That is, is there evidence of goal-directed behaviors on the part of the child through the use of eye gaze, pointing, showing or other gestures, with or without vocalizations? This is crucial because we assume that these behaviors are precursors to oral expression of intent. If they are present, we are usually somewhat less concerned about the appropriateness of the child's rate of language acquisition. If they are absent, we become more concerned. According to Bates (1976), children's early intentional communication attempts could be described as use of **protodeclaratives** and **protoimperatives** with one designed to use objects to get the attention of an adult and the other for using adults to help them get an object. In the case of the protodeclaratives, they should "grow up" to become statements/comments, for example, "That bear is fuzzy"; whereas protoimperatives should "grow up" to become request forms, for example, "Dad, get me that truck." As Owens (2001) pointed out, children who signal intent have clearly moved from the dyad to the triad stage where objects join the child and the "other" in a communication act.

Clinical Insight

Real word use involves the meeting of three criteria: (1) the child's production should sound like an approximation of a word in the language the child is learning, (2) it should be phonetically consistent, and (3) it should be produced in consistent contexts. If one or more of these criteria is missing, the child is producing a protoword form and not a real word. Clearly, however, the child is demonstrating gains in the right direction as he or she adds forms that possess at least two of these criteria.

One issue that has muddied the waters and left many researchers and clinicians concerned with regard to the normative data we do have at our disposal is the fact that the populations selected for sampling language behaviors have not always appropriately cut across socioeconomic, dialectal, racial, or ethnic lines and so the normative data available are frequently skewed to reflect the performances of children in the mainstream culture: white, middle-class speakers of Standard English (SE) dialect. There is no reason to assume that children from nonmainstream populations would demonstrate different rates of growth in terms of structures shared by dialects, but in the absence of supportive data, it may remain an open question for some and a source of misdiagnosis for others. Another related question has been that of providing practitioners with developmental data that have been based on a sufficient number of subjects to be meaningful. Although the database has been added to in recent years, note that Brown's original longitudinal Mean Length of Utterance (MLU) data were collected from the samples of three children. Moreover, the initial staging of syntax development according to MLU development was also based on this limited data set.

Even within the population of children who are learning SE, there have been some concerns that the children selected for study have not represented a cross-section of the different **language-learning styles** representing normal language acquisition. Nelson (1973) made this point in her studies of children's early vocabulary acquisition. She noted that the majority of children selected for her study were highly intelligible, discrete word users (that is, they did not show a predisposition for the use of formulas like "gimmedat") who tended to demonstrate a high proportion of nouns in their early vocabularies (greater than 50%) but this pattern did not describe all of the children in her study. This point is important because it emphasizes the fact that, even within the group of children viewed as normal language learners, there may be differences in styles of language learning. By styles we mean that different learning patterns may emerge, perhaps with different propensities for certain structures, but they ultimately appear to lead the child to the same point of adequate language competencies. Thus, no one style is presumed to be better than any other at this time. It also remains an open question as to whether there may not be additional as yet unidentified language-learning styles.

Clinical Insight

In discussions of language-learning style, it is also important to consider the impact of high-context versus low-context cultures. In high-context cultures, which represent the nonmainstream culture in the United States, children learn to focus in on the emphasis placed on nonlinguistic information and observational learning. Low-context learners are those who rely on the verbal message itself and less on the context in which it was presented (see Paul, 1995, p. 160, for a comparison of the two). A learning style resulting from exposure to low-context culture leads to a child's acceptance of decontextualized language lessons where clinician and child sit side-by-side, looking at the same materials and the clinician asks the child, "What's this?" For the child whose learning style is represented by the high-context culture, such an activity may appear to be odd (for an adult to be asking a child something the adult already knows).

Clinicians who work with the preschool-age population and must make judgments about the adequacy of their language acquisition need to remain actively cognizant of the fact that the normative data provided not only represent ranges of normalcy but also may be culturally as well as style-biased. It is necessary, therefore, for the speech-language clinician to be a careful consumer of normative data by determining the characteristics of the sample population used in any normative study or assessment tool and by carefully comparing it with her or his client. Fortunately, in the last several years there has been some improvement in the multicultural and multidialectal acquisition and use data available. Articles by Washington and Craig (1994) and Craig and Washington (1994) have provided some of the recent acquisition data for child speakers of AAE. In addition, Dr. Harry Seymour and his colleagues at the University of Massachusetts are currently at work on several projects designed to yield more normative data for young speakers learning AAE as well as designing a nonbiased, dialect-sensitive test for use with speakers of AAE (Seymour, 2000).

AN ILLUSTRATION OF NORMAL LANGUAGE DEVELOPMENT

> *When I think about what a preschool language disorder is NOT, I think first of my young friend, Joseph, at a time when he was not much more than 3 years of age. After 2 weeks of incessant and progressively more creative attempts on my part to convince him that it would be okay for him to accompany me to see "The Lion King" movie without his mother, I finally managed to convince him. He agreed to go with me—alone—without Mom, who had already seen it once and who was not up for seeing it again. "Great," I said to Joseph. "It's a date!" And he replied, "Okay. I do not drive, though."*

At the very most, this anecdote is funny because it describes a child who at age 3 demonstrated a somewhat sophisticated concept of the term "date," one with a number of social rules or expectations attached to it, expectations far beyond what he at age 3 knew he could deliver. This tells us something about this child's semantic repertoire as well as his pragmatic knowledge. At a less remarkable level, it describes a child who is attempting to maintain a topic introduced by his conversation partner and he managed to do so by adding some relevant information. In other words, Joe knows something about how to keep a conversation going and he has some strategies for doing so, if the topic is something he is familiar with. Notice that, to accomplish this, he has to draw on what he knows about the following language parameters:

* ❖ **Semantics**—the component of language that relates to a child's conceptual development, his world knowledge, vocabulary building, and the meaningful relationships that hold between words in a sentence, for example, Mommy go → agent + action (see Owens, 1996, p. 262, Table 8.7).

* ❖ **Syntax**—the component of language that deals with word order and the rule-governed combinations of words used to form grammatical sentences, for example, declaratives, interrogatives, and imperatives.

* ❖ **Morphology**—the portion of language that deals with the learning and use of meaningful units that can stand alone (whole words or *free morphemes*, e.g., house, tall) or serve as suffixes or prefixes (*bound morphemes*, e.g., 's, -ed) that enable children to express verb tense or noun number.

❖ **Pragmatics**—the portion of language that refers to the different ways we can use language according to differences in social contexts, such as communicative intentions (or functions), and conversation rules. Last, it was his ability in the area of:

❖ **Phonology**—the child's knowledge of the sound inventory of his or her language and the rules governing acceptable, that is, grammatical, combinations of those sounds into words, that permitted him to produce an intelligible sentence that I understood and made me giggle.

By age 3, Joe had managed to put a lot of the language development puzzle together. Not only were his receptive (e.g., understanding, language comprehension) and expressive (e.g., production) vocabularies growing on a daily basis but so was his ability to construct a variety of sentence types, such as questions and declaratives; his understanding of how to appropriately use the language he knows in a variety of social contexts; and the sound system of his first language was approaching the organization of that observed in adults speaking the same language.

In addition to the attention paid to Joe's ability to produce language accurately and appropriately, we know that his ability to understand the language he hears in the world around him is also developing. Of course, Joe has not completed his semantic concept of "date" yet, but there will be plenty of time for that in the years to come! Note, however, that through some exposure to this word, he has developed some rudimentary understanding of its meaning. A series of recent studies by Rice and her colleagues (see Oetting, Rice, & Swank, 1995, for example) has provided us with a good basis of knowledge about **fast mapping**, a child's ability to learn conceptual information from limited exposures, perhaps only one exposure, to new words in context. It represents one way of describing the child's strategy for learning new concepts. All of these aspects of Joe's language development, semantics, syntax, morphology, phonology, and pragmatics, will be the features of language we will want to analyze for the child suspected of a preschool language disorder and suggestions for doing so will be presented in the Procedures section.

The term **mapping** is also an important term. My preferred way of describing language learning to students and caregivers alike is that what children attempt to do is map, or connect up, the words they hear onto the actions and activities they observe. We will keep that in mind for the intervention portion of this guide where we talk about how to help make changes in a child's language acquisition process. One of these ways will be to facilitate the ability of the child to more successfully "map" by making the connections more obvious. So this means it will be important to provide language input that follows the activities at hand, using the context the child appears to be most focused on.

HOW DO LANGUAGE COMPONENT PARTS FIT TOGETHER?

In 1978, Bloom and Lahey presented their classic delineation of language form (e.g., syntax, morphology, phonology), from language content (e.g., semantics), and language use (e.g., pragmatics), explaining how in the normally developing child these component parts are developing at the same time and of necessity intersect or interact with one another. Their model depicts the now-famous three rings that perfectly intersect, creating the image of complementary functioning of the three aspects of language. How can this "complementizing" actually be observed? In one example that I particularly appreciate, Campbell and Shriberg (1982) noted that, when their subjects who had multiple speech sound errors were attempting to convey new information to their listeners, they were more likely to produce accurate productions of their "error" sounds. Thus pragmatics, the use of language in context making oneself understood in conversation, was having a positive effect on these children's phonology, in particular, the accuracy of the sounds selected for use within words that were more essential to the communication focus of the utterance.

Using their model, Bloom and Lahey (1978) also conceptualized that if any one or more of these components lagged behind the others in development to a significant degree, a language disorder resulted. Thus, a child may recognize the reciprocal, turn-taking nature of conversations (language use) but be unable to sufficiently mobilize his or her skills with language form to participate in that conversation with more than one word at a time. Or, a child may be facile at stringing words together into sentences (language form) but may be unable to produce any meaningful text in the process (language content).

Clinical Insight

Not all persons interested in describing the process of language learning necessarily see language form, content, and use as being equal partners in acquisition as Bloom and Lahey (1978) conceptualized. For some individuals, language *use* takes precedence over the other two. That is to say that these "Functionalists" believe that the language learning process may be driven by the need to communicate so that language use is the underlying, motivating factor determining what is learned and when (Bates & MacWhinney, 1982).

Prutting (1979) presented a model somewhat similar to Bloom and Lahey's (1978) when she described the language development of preschoolers in the areas of morphology/syntax, semantics, and phonology as a synergistic developmental process that was only artificially divided up into the separate components I have been discussing. And that is a very important point to remember. We divide up the language "pie" to talk about differences in the language-learning profiles we observe in our clients sometimes at the expense of seeing the Big Picture, which in this case involves the interactive nature of language components and the overall communicative success possible for our young clients.

So, whether it is language form that lags behind, or language use or language content, or combinations of two or all three, the outcome is a negative effect on the child's ability to communicate. When we consider preschool language disorders, it is important to think more globally than the child's competencies in the specific language components themselves. Instead, we ought to think about the child's ability to use those components in consort to communicate ideas and understand the communication bids of others. Fey's 1986 text *Language Intervention with Young Children* presents an intervention strategy based on this perspective that focuses on children's propensity for producing unsolicited conversation bids (assertives, such as comments or requests) and responding to the conversation bids of others (responsives, such as responses to a clarification request or a request for action). This model will be discussed in more detail in the Procedures section to follow.

WHAT SHOULD WE LOOK FOR WHEN OBSERVING CHILDREN'S COMMUNICATION COMPETENCE?

Some specific, important things to consider concerning the child's communication ability are as follows. While we are observing preschool-age children, it will be important to ask ourselves some basic questions about the child's more general ability to communicate. For example, can the child meet the communication demands placed on him or her at home or in his or her day care setting or in preschool environments? That is, is the child able to use the language competencies that he or she possesses to learn from the world? When necessary, does the child ask for clarification in the classroom? Or, is the child able to follow along in conversations with his or her classmates as part of play routines? So, it is commonly believed today that, in addition to our careful analyses of the specific linguistic, utterance level, phenomena observed in the preschool child's repertoire, we should pay careful attention to the more general or macrolevel communication abilities of the child. How does the child use these utterances to form conversation structures?

It may also be the case that we will not collect all of this information ourselves. If a classroom teacher and staff are available who can serve as informed observers for a particular child, consulting with the appropriate person may obviate or greatly reduce the need for you to spend time directly in the classroom gathering this information.

That means that our evaluations will involve more than just what data we can derive from standardized testing, amassed in one setting and in one communication context. And, our treatment strategies are likely to involve more than just a therapy room for a setting and a speech-language clinician as the provider of language-learning opportunities. The use of standardized testing also continues to be a controversial area in the evaluation of the language of preschool-age children (see Lund & Duchan, 1993, for a perspective on testing in more natural settings). Note that when we use standardized tests to investigate language use, we invariably are using highly decontextualized materials and situations. How, then, do we expect the child to give us a representative sample of the way he or she typically uses language if we take away the naturalness of the situation? Suggestions for dealing with the issue of naturalness will be also be presented in the Procedures section that deals with assessment and treatment.

Regardless of the method(s) we choose for assessment, and keeping in mind the cautions previously delineated, it will still be critical to have some information documenting the normal expectations for development.

Some Special References for Normative Data Regarding Language Development

A number of user-friendly resources exist for providing the normative developmental data that clinicians need to have at their fingertips. Here are three that I have found to be quite useful.

   1. Kent, R. (1994). *Reference manual for communicative sciences and disorders: Speech and language.* Austin, TX: Pro-Ed.

   This manual includes a plethora of reference tables and charts not only focusing on language and communication development (Sections 1, 5, and 6), but also including some assessment protocols for nonstandardized assessment. The tables and charts included have been culled from a variety of published sources. I have found this volume to be a real time saver, and on more than one occasion when I have consulted it, I have found exactly what I needed and even more than I thought was available.

2. Retherford-Stickler, K. (1996). NCA: *Normal communication acquisition: An animated database of behaviors* (CD-ROM). Eau Claire, WI: Thinking Publications.

   This CD-ROM is summarized by the author as a "database of developmental behaviors from birth to age 12 years and beyond. The user may search the database by developmental component. Each entry includes examples and research citation." I personally have found the animated sequences the least useful portion of this resource. The tables and charts, however, provide a quick and easy reference to a number of highly useful and up-to-date developmental charts suitable for in-clinic use to illustrate for caregivers, classroom teachers, and other professionals the progression of normal language learning.

3. Owens, R. (2001). *Language development: An introduction* (5th ed.). Needham Heights, MA: Allyn & Bacon.

   This basic text on language development provides the reader with a comprehensive but readable compilation of current information about how normally developing children learn language. There is a liberal inclusion of tables and figures for summary of important taxonomies used in the study of child language.

ETIOLOGIES OF LANGUAGE DISORDER IN PRESCHOOL CHILDREN

Getting back to my friend Joseph, why has he been so lucky in terms of his burgeoning language-learning prowess? We have a set of general assumptions:

❖ He has the necessary cognitive prerequisites for language learning, including the ability to discriminate between similar stimuli and distinguish between what is familiar and what is unfamiliar, to generalize, and to organize information into categories that facilitate retrieval of information, and

❖ adequate hearing for receiving the speech signals critical for both language comprehension and production development at the phonetic as well as conversational levels.

❖ We also assume that his social-behavioral development is sufficiently normal so that Joseph is motivated to learn and then use language to communicate in conventional ways with the people in his environment. There are some children who may have figured out how to use the communication code but who prefer not to frequently display the skills they have. For these children, the role of temperament may come into play. Developmentally, some children seem to focus in on one area of developmental learning at a time or discover that, for them, physical interactions and thus motor learning is easier or sufficiently expressive or both. Some children just have a quieter or more reserved style of interaction.

❖ We also assume that Joseph's neurological system is intact so that he can rely on the use of his body for linguistic or nonlinguistic expression whether it is the innervation of his articulators that he uses to produce speech sounds, or his arms and fingers to gesture, or his lips and facial musculature to smile and indicate acknowledgment instead of saying "okay."

❖ Overall, there is the assumption that Joseph's genetic makeup played a role in sealing his fate as a language-normal child.

Clinical Insight

Recent genetic studies have shown us rather convincingly that language disorders tend to cluster in families (Tallal, Ross, & Curtiss, 1989; Tomblin, 1989). In addition, Tomblin, Freese, and Records (1992) provided more convincing data to show that adults who showed evidence of SLI when they were children are very likely to continue to demonstrate symptoms of depressed language abilities. In particular, these studies have demonstrated a greater likelihood for language disorders to be present in the fathers and brothers of the children diagnosed with SLI than in their mothers or their sisters. Tomblin and his colleagues suggested that, for some children, a genetic cause for SLI is the likely predicting factor, but that genetics alone does not explain all cases of SLI. It is also possible, they noted, that, for some children, although the genetic "loading" is present, mitigating factors, such as an appropriately stimulating environment, compensate.

❖ In addition to all of the capabilities that it is commonly assumed Joseph must bring to the language-learning situation to ensure success, we also assume that his environment is providing him with a context conducive to language learning: lots of opportunities to experience others' use of both familiar and unfamiliar words and sentences and sentences turned into conversations (linguistic input) as well as opportunities for him to practice employing their use.

Clinical Insight

The input provided needs to be presented in such a way that the child is able to see the relationship between the words and the language context. As already noted, the child has to be able to "map," or connect, the language heard (or seen) to what he or she is observing in the outside world. These opportunities are most often provided by caregivers both inside and outside the family unit, some of whom may be quite naturally skilled in the provision of an appropriate language environment. If this were not the case, if our assumptions about Joseph were incorrect and he was unable to compensate for deficits in any of these areas and those deficits were significant enough, then it is quite possible that he would be demonstrating a language disorder rather than producing the normally developing language he so matter-of-factly uses in his activities of daily living.

WHAT IS A LANGUAGE DISORDER FROM THE PROFESSIONAL PERSPECTIVE?

Committees comprised of American Speech-Language-Hearing Association members with expertise in the area of language development and disorders have contributed to our collective understanding about the scope of language disorders and the acceptable paths to intervening with those disorders. In their 1983 definition of *language* developed by the Committee on Language, the American Speech-Language-Hearing Association was careful to point out that language is a dynamic and multifaceted phenomenon that includes the aspects of pragmatics, phonology, morphology, semantics, and syntax. The definition went on to include the proposal that language acquisition and its use evolve from a number of different factors acting in consort, or perhaps out of sync in the case of the child with a language disorder: cognitive, psychosocial, biological, and environmental. The notion that the primary purpose of language is communicative is also considered in this statement. Conveyed also is the sense that when we consider language competencies, we have to consider them within the broader context of human interaction. Note that this focus on a more general or conceptual, communicative level remains important more than 15 years later and is evident in many of the intervention programs aimed either at educating caregivers to better facilitate language learning (see Giralometto, Greenberg, & Manolson, 1986; MacDonald, 1989; Weiss, 1981) or aimed directly at making changes in their children's language behaviors that will be described in the Procedures section.

The 1983 Position Statement was followed by an ASHA 1988 technical report explicating the issues surrounding the determination of eligibility for language intervention, and these issues will also be discussed later in the Procedures section. The committee adopted a definition of language disorders borrowed from Bloom and Lahey (1978). Stating that they intended to use the term *language disorder* broadly, the committee *considered any individual child to be language disordered when his or her language competencies were different from those expected considering the child's chronological age.* Again, it should be remembered that we are considering both language comprehension and expression in this definition.

Clinical Insight

The use of chronological age as a determinant of language disorder versus mental age has been problematic for some clinical researchers. Another one of the controversies in the area of language disorders, specifically for SLI in preschoolers, is what Fey, Long, and Cleave (1994) refer to as an arbitrary cutoff of an IQ of greater than or equal to 85 as the determination point for exclusion from the SLI population.

Given this definition of a language disorder, we know that potentially there are a number of factors that could act on the process of language learning either singly or together to create problems.

❖ For example, we know that most children with a moderate to profound bilateral hearing loss, that is, a biological factor, who are attempting to learn oral language without amplification and/or specialized training, are going to have a very difficult time learning how to speak intelligibly. (Note that learning language does not require the adoption of an oral mode of expression and a primarily aural mode for input. Sign language is as viable a form of language as any other, although it can be argued that signed language is not used as universally as oral communication.)

❖ Similarly, the child with a significant cognitive deficit might be expected to experience difficulties in language learning as would

❖ The antisocial child exhibiting bizarre, self-stimulating behaviors who does not appear capable of recognizing conversation let alone how to take part in it and who may be diagnosed as functioning on the spectrum of autistic disorders, and

❖ Children with significant mobility or motor planning disorders that inhibit their ability to communicate intelligibly (developmental apraxia of speech) or explore their world (cerebral palsy).

What I have described here are purer cases of etiology and often in practice they will be anything but that "clean." In situations where an etiology can be established early or at least suggested from deficits noted in hearing ability, social-emotional development, or cognitive development, the term *language disorder* is appropriate. And, much has been written about the special difficulties in language learning encountered by the child with a hearing impairment learning oral speech and language, or children diagnosed as performing in the severely mentally retarded range, or children diagnosed with autism, and so forth. Note, too, that with each different etiology of preschool language disorder treatment may be somewhat different, just as treatment is not the same for all individuals with voice problems or adults with language difficulties. But this guide is not about children who have a language disorder whose origin can be more easily identified by these etiologies. There will be separate guides to tackle those types of language disorders. Instead, this guide will focus on the type of language disorder that appears to exist in the absence of a hearing impairment, IQ deficiency, motor problems, or social-emotional impairment. It is most commonly referred to in the literature as SLI (Bishop & Edmundson, 1987; Conti-Ramsden, Crutchley, & Botting, 1997; Leonard, 1998; Stark & Tallal, 1981; Watkins & Rice, 1994).

HOW PREVALENT A PROBLEM IS SLI?

According to the results of the 1997 Omnibus Survey conducted by the American Speech-Language-Hearing Association, approximately 8% of the speech-language pathologists and audiologists responding spend the greatest part of their day working in a preschool setting, although a much larger proportion, 72%, reported that they regularly serve some children who are diagnosed with "other childhood language disorders." It is assumed from the other options given in the survey that this category was used for children diagnosed with SLI. When asked about the percentage of preschoolers (ages 3 to 5) in their typical monthly caseload, the same responders revealed that 15% of their caseload fit into this age range.

The National Institute of Deafness and Other Communication Disorders (NIDCD) (1995) reported that approximately 8 to 12% of preschool-age children demonstrate a language impairment of some form and that many of these children will be labeled as SLI, more specifically about 5% of preschoolers will meet the criteria for SLI. Their findings also supported a gender bias for the disorder, with males more often fitting the diagnosis of SLI than females at a 2:1 margin. A more recent epidemiologic study focusing on the prevalence of SLI in kindergarten-age children completed by Tomblin and his associates (1997) yielded a prevalence rate of 7.4% of the population when using a Performance Scale IQ criterion of 85 or higher. If a lower cutoff point for nonverbal IQ is used for a criterion, an additional 5% of the population examined by Tomblin, Records, Buckwalter, Zhang, Smith, and O'Brien (1997) would fall into the category of SLI yielding a total of 12% of kindergarten-age children. In this study, however, no significant difference in inclusion by gender was observed. In any event, when percentages of children affected by SLI are considered, it is clear that SLI is not a trivial problem.

Another important finding of the most recent ASHA Omnibus Survey (1997) was that a majority of speech-language pathologists and audiologists rated the availability of professional resources in the area of specific language disorders as good or excellent. Judging by the large number of research articles in recent issues of the *Journal of Speech, Language and Hearing Research* devoted to SLI, not only are clinicians facing the challenge of the child diagnosed with SLI on their caseloads, but researchers are devoting considerable energy to determining how to best characterize SLI, how to best evaluate it, and how to best treat it.

HOW IS SLI DETERMINED?

As noted by Watkins (1994, p. 2), classically SLI has been a disorder of exclusion rather than inclusion. This is a recurring theme in the literature. That is, children have been described by the characteristics they are not exhibiting rather than those they are exhibiting. These children are not demonstrating hearing losses, cognitive deficits, neurological deficits, or social-emotional problems. If they are, then the etiology for the language disorder is generally placed at the feet of that problem.

The first standard definition of SLI was proposed by Stark and Tallal in 1981 to assist researchers in selecting comparable populations of children for study (for an excellent and exhaustive review of the history of SLI, see Leonard, 1998) and it contained the following criteria:

❖ First, the child's standardized test scores for language yielded age equivalents of one year lower than the child's chronological age (CA) or mental age (MA).

❖ The child must *also* demonstrate each of the following:

  1. Hearing thresholds must fall within normal limits (not greater than 25 dB).

  2. The child's Performance IQ (nonverbal testing) falls within ± one standard deviation of the mean. For most studies this will mean a score of 85 or higher.

  3. There has been no report by a parent, teacher, or other caregiver of the presence of an emotional/behavioral problem that would interfere with language learning.

  4. The child does not exhibit a severe or profound speech sound disorder that interferes with intelligibility.

  5. The child shows no evidence of having significant neurological deficits.

❖ If any of these five criteria are not met, the child is excluded from this definition of SLI.

DO SUBGROUPINGS OF SLI CHILDREN EXIST?

Other investigators have described delineations of the characteristics of groups of children with SLI. This information is important for practicing clinicians to know about for the purposes of appropriate diagnosis and treatment planning as well as to have a historical perspective regarding the evolution of thinking about this disorder. When researchers have identified subgroupings of children with SLI, they have usually had the hopes of identifying differential paths and rates to recovery.

In 1987 Rapin and Allen speculated that six possible subgroupings for children with SLI might better describe the diversity of the disorder:

❖ lexical syntactic deficit syndrome

❖ verbal auditory agnosia

❖ verbal dyspraxia

❖ phonological programming deficit syndrome

❖ phonological-syntactic deficit syndrome

❖ semantic-pragmatic deficit syndrome.

In a later paper, Rapin (1996) noted that these six subgroupings probably could be consolidated into three groups without sacrificing any of their diagnostic power:

❖ expressive language disorders

❖ expressive-receptive language disorder

❖ higher-order processing disorders

Similarly, Conti-Ramsden and her colleagues (1997) delineated three subgroupings of children with SLI, referring to them as:

❖ expressive SLI

❖ expressive-receptive SLI

❖ complex SLI (i.e., children who demonstrated problems learning lexical, syntactic, semantic, and pragmatic competencies but had no phonological component to the disorder.)

Conti-Ramsden and her colleagues (1997) concluded that as a group the children who had been diagnosed as demonstrating SLI from whom they had collected their data continued to show the same basic configurations of subgroup characteristics over time. However, individual children were lacking in stability. That is, within the group an individual child's relative language strengths and weaknesses would be likely to change over time. The authors concluded that SLI was a "dynamic condition" (p. 1204) and, this being the case, suggested that it was then also likely to be positively affected by intervention. Earlier, Bishop and Edmundson (1987) had noted that approximately 37% of the children they had studied who had been diagnosed with SLI by age 4 were no longer performing like children with SLI when they reached age 5½.

More recently, Tomblin provided a cautionary note with regard to subtyping in SLI. He suggested that children who demonstrate SLI whose primary problem is in expressive language learning, may be overrepresented versus their proportion in the population of children with SLI as a whole. These are the children most likely to be considered to have problems by parents and other professionals. Although the group of children with receptive difficulties *only* may be relatively small, they, in turn, may be the ones over-looked by families and clinicians because their difficulties are so much more subtle than the problems of children with expressive delays. This may also explain why the major-ity of the children originally labeled as having SLI at age 5 by Tomblin's research group (Tomblin et al., 1997) who were enrolled in therapy, were receiving therapy for speech sound disorders only by the time they had reached the second grade (Weiss, Buckwalter, Tomblin, & Zhang, 1999).

WHAT IS THE RELATIONSHIP BETWEEN "LATE TALKERS" AND SLI?

The child who is late to begin talking, both in terms of acquisition of first words and pro-duction of first word combinations, may be at particular risk for the development of SLI. The proportions often discussed are between 25 to 50% of children diagnosed as "late talkers" eventually are diagnosed as SLI. Due to the variability in developmental course, Leonard (1998) has suggested that a diagnosis of SLI prior to age 3 is not yet a possi-bility. However, several groups of researchers have studied children who have been identified by various sets of criteria as "late talkers" and when followed longitudinally some indeed fulfilled the diagnostic criteria of SLI by the time they had reached their third birthdays. Given that not all children thus identified around age 2 go on to be classified as SLI, there must be some differences within this group of children that can help differentially predict their likelihood for SLI diagnosis. This is one of the questions that drives research with "late talkers."

Rate of vocabulary development and use of communicative gestures have been the prime language behavior data collected in studies of "late talkers." Criteria for labeling as a "late talker" has varied somewhat from research group to research group. For example, Rescorla (1989) considered any child who had reached his or her second birth-day with an expressive vocabulary of less than 50 different single words and without any word combinations as a "late talker." For another series of studies, Paul (1991) considered children between 18 and 23 months of age to be "late talkers" if they were not producing at least 10 different single words. "Late talkers" have also been shown to demonstrate less mature development of their phonological systems (Rescorla & Bernstein Ratner, 1996), symbolic play behaviors (Rescorla & Goosens, 1992), and limited socialization skills (Paul, Spangle-Looney, & Dahm, 1991) when compared with age-matched, normally developing peers.

Some of the major findings from longitudinal studies of "late talkers" that have addressed prognosis are:

❖ Children who demonstrated reduced receptive as well as expressive compe-tencies were more likely to continue to experience language delays than children whose comprehension abilities were normal but demonstrated expressive language delays (Thal, Tobias, & Morrison, 1991).

❖ When children diagnosed as "late talkers" have both comprehension and production delays, they are five times more likely to have a family member who has a history of a language-learning disorder (Paul & Unkefer, 1995, in Leonard, 1998).

❖ Two-year-old "late-talking" children who were more likely to catch up with their peers by age 3, were children who utilized gestures to enhance their limited verbal output (Thal et al., 1991).

❖ Paul and Smith (1993) found that their 4-year-old subjects, diagnosed as "late talkers," who persisted in use of immature syntax, were also likely to show reduced abilities to form narratives and had lexicons that were less diverse than those of their normally developing peers.

❖ Whitehurst and his colleagues (Whitehurst, Fischel, Arnold, & Lonigan, 1992) followed a group of "late talkers" from approximately 2½ to 5½ years of age in terms of their vocabulary growth. They noted a steady decrease in percentage of children failing to reach the normal range of performance on two vocabulary measures over those three years of development. Although approximately half of the children failed to reach the normal range of performance on one or the other of the tests by age 3, that percentage had dropped to less than 10% by the end of the study.

As Leonard (1998) noted, the Whitehurst data and other data collected by Paul and her colleagues that point to a significant proportion of "late talkers" catching up with their age-matched peers by the time they reach the early school years should not suggest that early intervention is not a useful and clinically appropriate endeavor with this population.

GIVEN THE DIFFERENT DELINEATIONS OF SLI SUBGROUPS, ARE THERE ANY CHARACTERISTICS THAT TRANSCEND THESE?

In addition to not demonstrating any of the expected deficits that are usually closely associated with language disorder, several specific characteristics of this group of children have been delineated. This has become another recurring theme in the literature. That is, in addition to providing exclusion criteria, what are the patterns of behavior that children classified as SLI do exhibit? As noted by Watkins (1994) in Watkins and Rice (1994), research has demonstrated at least three features that appear to be shared by children diagnosed as SLI:

❖ There is a great deal of variability of language performance within the population. This heterogeneity can affect the severity of the language problem, the area of language affected, and the modality or modalities affected. Thus, we know that, although learning grammatical morphology is often the most severely affected of the areas of language learning, SLI can manifest itself in other areas or combinations of language areas, for example, semantics and pragmatics. A child may show a pattern of uniform depression in language learning across areas or modalities, that is, comprehension and/or expression, or the profile may show more individual differentiation, with adequate comprehension skills but a significant deficit in expressive language, for example.

❖ We also know that children diagnosed with SLI are likely to demonstrate social interactive problems (see Rice, 1993, for a review of this literature) that manifest themselves later as conversational and other pragmatic deficits (see Brinton & Fujiki, 1989; 1995). One reason for this is that children with poorer language skills are often not preferred playmates or may be avoided altogether by their classroom peers. This means that children with SLI are given fewer opportunities for conversational interaction to practice what they may know about language as well as receive sufficient up-close-and-personal peer modeling. In the intervention portion of the Procedures section of the guide, you will find information about Fey's (1986) assertiveness-responsiveness continuum and how children with SLI who understand and can enact both of their roles in conversation are believed by the author to have the best prognosis of all because they are able to create their own language-learning opportunities.

❖ There is sufficient literature to suggest that the problem of SLI is ongoing. That is, children diagnosed with SLI by the time they are in kindergarten are more likely to demonstrate problems learning to read and write (see Catts & Kamhi, 1998, for a review of the connections between language learning and success in learning literacy skills). In 1980, Snyder suggested that many of our dismissals of kindergarten-age children from therapy were premature because we were likely to see them back in treatment once reading and writing are being taught. She further suggested that we may be failing to teach them the preliteracy skills they need to know, like inferencing and phonological awareness, to lay the foundation for successful reading and writing. More recently, Snow, Burns, and Griffin (1998) in their edited summary of the literature on predicting reading disabilities noted that the presence of a language disorder diagnosed prior to kindergarten was a major predictor of later difficulties in learning to read.

In a recent epidemiological study of the prevalence of SLI in kindergarten children (Tomblin et al., 1997), the investigators used the following set of criteria to identify their SLI population. First, potential subjects were excluded if there was historical evidence of mental retardation, neurological problems, or autism. The child then needed to pass either a pure-tone screening or, subsequent to failing a pure-tone screening, a threshold test and tympanometry (see Tomblin et al., 1997, pp. 1250–1251 for details), demonstrate a Performance Scale IQ greater than 85, and fail two or more of the five composite language scores yielded from selected subtests of the *Test of Language Development-2:P* (*TOLD-2P*; Newcomer & Hammill, 1992) and a test of narrative comprehension and one of story recall. Failure was set at −1.25 standard deviations from the mean score at the child's chronological age level. See Tomblin, Records, and Zhang (1996) for an explanation of how these composite scores were derived and the rationale for their use.

In terms of the etiology of SLI, other researchers have explored the possibility that at the base of SLI is the child's difficulty with processing rapid auditory information. This is the line of research and speculation that Tallal and her colleagues have pursued through the development of their controversial FastForword training program (Merzenich, Jenkins, Johnston, Schreiner, Miller, & Tallal, 1996). There has been considerable controversy spawned by the preliminary reports of the success of this program. Many of these concerns have surrounded the selective presentation of the outcome data and the standardized tests used to evaluate student progress. See Rice's (1997) and Tallal's (1997) opposing commentaries about the interpretations of the preliminary findings of this approach.

Still others have viewed SLI as having something to do with poor skills at subtle aspects of nonverbal cognitive abilities that are not discerned by available performance

IQ tests. That is, these children may have difficulty manipulating symbols; for example, one study demonstrated that children with SLI have difficulties with tasks involving mental rotation (Johnson & Ellis Weismer, 1983). Studies that have compared children labeled as SLI with same-age peers have also shown that the children with SLI demonstrate less well-developed symbolic play abilities (Brown, Redmond, Liebergott, & Swope, 1975).

And there are still others who view SLI not as a product of deficits in what the child brings to the language-learning environment but as a result of the impoverished language-learning environment in which the child spends his or her days. That is, if we believe that some minimum quality and quantity of language input is needed for the learning of the language system, it can be the case that some children are not getting their requirements. When this occurs, the child learns an abbreviated language repertoire or is at least delayed in its acquisition. Unfortunately, we do not know what the minimums are. Given the overwhelming number of children who learn language without any difficulty, we can assume that most children are receiving enough linguistic input from a variety of sources. It is when there are language-learning difficulties that we are often stuck in determining whether one factor is a depressed amount of language input. It may be that children with language-learning problems require a greater amount of language input and a more specialized type of language input, perhaps slower and more repetitive, because their ability to make the most of any input they do receive is poor at best.

As noted earlier, the most likely type of language difficulty experienced by the child with SLI is in learning the use of grammatical morphemes and the underlying reason for this difficulty has generated a good deal of research and controversy in the last several years in the fields of psychology and linguistics as well as in speech pathology and audiology. There have been at least three hypotheses put forth in the literature lately to attempt to explain this phenomenon. Leonard, Eyer, Bedore, and Grela (1997) provide a succinct description of the three:

❖ The "extended optional infinitive" approach studied by Rice, Wexler, and their associates (see Rice & Wexler, 1995), assumes that children with SLI persist in leaving verbs in main clauses unmarked, which is a pattern frequently seen in younger, normally developing children who appear for a time to lack the recognition when tense marking is obligatory.

❖ The "implicit rule deficit" approach proposed by Gopnik and colleagues (see Gopnik & Crago, 1991), suggests that the individual with SLI cannot generalize rule formulations based on verb tense and subject number, for example, so that the rule systems that are formed rather automatically in the language development of the normally developing child does not find the same underlying support in the child with SLI.

❖ The "surface" approach proposed by Leonard and his colleagues (Leonard, McGregor, & Allen, 1992), which focuses on the processing demands placed on the young child to correctly use English grammatical morphemes, where morphemes that are brief in duration or unstressed in presentation present the most difficulty for children with SLI.

Recently, Leonard, Eyer, Bedore, and Grela (1997) attempted to test each of these hypotheses to see if one or more could serve as a reasonable explanation for these frequently observed difficulties with the learning of grammatical morphemes. The investigators used a data set collected from preschool-age children exhibiting SLI and a matched group of controls, specifically children who were younger than the group of children with SLI but who demonstrated the same Mean Length of Utterance (MLU), a measure of utterance length and complexity based on the average number of morphemes per utterance (Brown, 1973). Their results revealed support for two of the hypotheses, specifically the "surface" approach and the "extended optional infinitive" approach but did not show evidence that would uphold the expected outcome of the "implicit rule deficit" approach to explaining SLI and problems with grammatical morphemes. Leonard et al. (1997) noted that the "surface" explanation may have greater applicability across morphemes than the "extended optional infinitive" explanation, as the latter does a good job of predicting problems with tense markers but a less sufficient job with other types of morphemes.

What we are left with for the most part are several theories of why SLI exists at all and several explanations for why and how it manifests itself as it does in the language repertoires of those who are diagnosed with it. It may be that no one unifying theory will ever explain all of the children who fit the definition of SLI. What we do know for certain, however, is that the problem of children diagnosed with SLI is a very real one. The numbers suggest that not only is there a sizable population of youngsters fitting these diagnostic criteria, but that there are many speech-language clinicians already called upon to provide language habilitation or rehabilitation services for them. We are still in the process of determining the types of service delivery models and specific treatment approaches that are the most efficacious for them.

Most troubling may be the observation that many preschool-age children with SLI go on to become the school-age children who have difficulty learning to read and write and remain burdened with some level of language impairment for the rest of their lives in a majority culture that has a tendency to reward those who are not only literate but who can communicate well. Is it a question of identifying these children earlier, and providing appropriate intervention services early on to prevent the blossoming of a full-blown language disorder? Or, given the possibility of a genetically determined disorder, is habilitation or rehabilitation even a reasonable goal? These are very legitimate questions, especially when they are directed at the SLP by family members of the preschool-age child diagnosed with SLI. To date, we know that some children will make clinically significant gains while others remain with lifelong language deficits of varying degrees. The challenge will be to determine which child without intervention is likely to be which as early as possible and this will involve painstaking research employing methods that are longitudinal, as well as retrospective and cross-sectional.

One phenomenon that can be troubling for clinicians and caregivers alike was described by Scarborough and Dobrich (1990) as "illusory recovery." This refers to an observed pattern in the treatment of young children with language disorders. Specifically, the authors noted that preschoolers who have received language treatment for their language disorders may test within the normal range around the time they are about to enter kindergarten and be dismissed from therapy, only to have their language difficulties reemerge when literacy learning becomes the focus of their first and second grade academic work. The authors explain this pattern by suggesting that there is a natural plateauing in language learning around 5 years of age so the child with an early language disorder may appear to catch up. Unfortunately, this plateau ends for normally developing children shortly thereafter when reading and writing skills are usually first taught. The child with the underlying language deficit once again exhibits difficulties with the processing and formulation of language symbols, this time with written symbols. The moral of this story is to approach early dismissal from treatment for the preschool-age child with some caution and skepticism. Consideration of monitoring the child's ability to maintain his or her language competencies in the absence of regularly scheduled treatment is always a good idea, so that, if the "illusion" of normalcy changes, it will be more likely that the child can be reinstated into treatment without too much delay. It would also be prudent to let parents and other caregivers know about the longevity of many language disorders so that they are not completely taken by surprise should their child need to return to speech-language services.

WHAT DO WE KNOW ABOUT *OTHER* GENERAL LANGUAGE CHARACTERISTICS OF PRESCHOOL-AGE CHILDREN DIAGNOSED WITH SLI?

Basically, there is evidence to suggest that delays and differences in acquisition rate and performance exist in all areas of language for most children with SLI.

❖ **Pragmatic Development:** Because of their limitations in learning the morphology and syntax of their language, some children with SLI have been shown to be limited in their ability to express a number of different communicative intentions. However, it is not clear that these children did not underlyingly have these language functions in their repertoires (Fey, Leonard, Fey, & O'Connor, 1978). That is, many children with SLI have been shown to rely on gestures and stereotypic phrases to convey specific language functions. In terms of SLI children's abilities with conversation participation, they have appeared to be less able than normally developing children to enter into ongoing conversations (Craig & Washington, 1993). Although they do not appear to have the strategies, linguistic or otherwise, to do this, they do much better when they are involved in dyadic conversation interactions. Gallagher and Darnton (1978) noted that, although children with SLI recognized the need to make clarifications in their messages when requested to do so by their listeners, they were less likely than younger, normally developing children to have a complete repertoire of strategies for doing so.

❖ **Vocabulary/Semantic Development:** Children with SLI typically show slower acquisition of their first words and continue to show slower acquisition of new words into their lexicons. As Leonard (1998) pointed out, it is not the case that the child with SLI begins word learning at the appropriate age but just continues learning words at a slower pace. Instead, word learning is often delayed from the very start. This may prove to be an important feature to "flag" when interviewing caregivers about important developmental milestones. One way in which children with SLI begin to show a different pattern of development rather than merely a delayed one is in their demonstration of a more limited repertoire of verbs (Watkins, Rice, & Moltz, 1993) than was seen with either same-age matches or language-age matches. In studies that controlled the number of presentations of novel words to children described as SLI, more exposures to the novel words were necessary for these children to add the words to both their receptive and expressive vocabularies than it was for same-age peers (Rice, Buhr, & Oetting, 1992; Rice, Oetting, Marquis, Bode, & Poe, 1994). Word combinations are also slower to appear in children with diagnoses of SLI (Trauner, Wulfeck, Tallal, & Hesselink, 1995, in Leonard, 1998). Trauner et al. found an average age of 37 months for word combinations in their subjects with SLI as opposed to 17 months for their normally developing subjects, according to Leonard (1998).

❖ **Syntax Development**

- *Comprehension*: deficits in language comprehension for children with SLI have been borne out in a number of studies. Interestingly, Bishop (1979) found that children previously diagnosed as SLI but having only expressive language deficits demonstrated difficulties with both vocabulary comprehension and grammatical comprehension tasks when these children's performance was compared with that of controls.

- *Production*: A number of studies have investigated the syntactic structure used by preschool-age children diagnosed with SLI, comparing their performances with age-matched or language-matched children. Their results have fallen into two basic groups—those that showed restricted complexities of structure on the part of the children with SLI (Morehead & Ingram, 1973), or similar structures used, but used with considerably less frequency (Leonard, 1972). In the second section we will talk about evidence that appears to indicate that there are differential prognoses for children with deficits in both comprehension and production versus those with problems in comprehension only.

❖ **Phonological Development:** Children who present with depressed competencies in the areas of vocabulary and grammatical development are also likely to exhibit delays in learning the sound system of their language. Likewise, if a child's main problem is in the area of phonological development, there is a high degree of likelihood that problems with both language comprehension and production will also be observed (Shriberg & Kwiatkowski, 1994). According to Shriberg and Kwiatkowski (1994) these numbers are far from trivial: approximately 8 out of 10 children will show expressive language deficits and about one third will exhibit problems achieving age-expected language comprehension scores. One additional phonological hallmark of the child with SLI appears to be a higher than typical degree of phonetic variability (Grunwell, 1992). Additional studies that have looked at acquisition rates of speech sound segments, or the presence of phonological processes in the children's repertoires, have demonstrated a generally slower rate of acquisition than observed in normally developing children. Further, anecdotal reports of children with SLI have revealed what appear to be the incorporation of unusual or "nonnatural" phonological processes into their speech sound repertoires (Leonard & Leonard, 1985). Some researchers exclude children with significant phonological disorders from their definition of SLI.

So the message of this brief summary of research findings is that, while the child with SLI can almost always be counted on to demonstrate deficits in the acquisition of grammatical morphology, it is also apparent that language problems are likely to be manifested in some or all other language areas. And, although these deficits in language learning are likely to have a direct and negative effect on the child's ability to communicate, many different treatment approaches have demonstrated some success in enhancing the language skills of these youngsters.

Researchers in the area of language disorders are continuing to investigate the nature of language disorders with the hope of identifying earlier children who will have difficulties learning language. Therefore appropriate intervention can be provided sooner, helping to avoid secondary problems. Leonard (1998) continues his series of cross-linguistic studies casting a wider net for the answers. Longitudinal studies like those undertaken by Tomblin and his colleagues may be able to show us that, for some of these children, the course of intervention is a brief one; for others, deficits in the area of language disorders first identified during the preschool years may manifest themselves for a lifetime.

SECTION

PROCEDURES

∙ ∙

This section includes figures, lists, questionnaires, and procedures for the assessment and evaluation of the preschool-age child with a suspected language disorder. For children with diagnosed language disorders, procedures and protocols for intervention follow. The title of the topic will be listed along with answers to the following questions:

WHO? This response denotes for whom this topic is most relevant. Usually this will be all SLPs providing service to preschool-age children at-risk for or with diagnosed language disorders.

WHAT? This response will denote the theme of the topic (e.g., working with parents of children with language disorders).

WHY? Denotes the importance of the topic (e.g., to validly and reliably evaluate the child's ability to produce appropriate answers to a variety of Wh-questions).

HOW? Lists specific ways in which the topic can be carried out.

WHERE? Denotes special contextual information that may be helpful in choosing the setting for the procedure.

LITERATURE RESOURCES Lists resources that supply this information; delineates results from research studies that serve to provide a rationale for the topic.

ASSESSMENT AND EVALUATION

General Considerations

As all practicing clinicians are aware, there are several different purposes for assessment and evaluation (see Tomblin, Morris, & Spriestersbach, 1999, for a comprehensive explanation of the diagnostician's role). Certainly diagnosis is chief among them, although assessment and evaluation procedures play an important part in determining the amount of progress made by a child from one evaluation period to another and aid in selecting different intervention strategies. In this section suggestions are given about how SLPs go about answering the question: Is a language disorder present in this preschool-age child? All components of language will be considered from pragmatics through syntax, morphology, semantics, and phonology.

One issue that needs to be addressed first is the fact that many speech-language clinicians make a distinction between the terms *assessment* and *evaluation* whereas others make no distinction between the two terms and use them interchangeably. For some clinicians, assessment refers to the determination of the presence of a problem whereas evaluation refers to measuring the specific aspects of the child's competencies relative to age-level expectations. For still others, assessment relates to the nonstandardized, observational measures that speech-language clinicians may first apply when a language disorder is suspected and they then use the term *evaluation* as the term applied to the process that incorporates a standardized test battery, following the assessment that yielded evidence of a potential language disorder. In this resource guide, the terms *assessment* and *evaluation* are used interchangeably, thus the topics that might be separated out between the two, for example, nonstandardized and observational procedures versus standardized testing, are included under the more general heading of Assessment/Evaluation procedures.

Note, too, that when we are considering SLI the question will become somewhat more narrowly focused because what we will want to determine is whether the difficulties the child is experiencing are best described as SLI. This being the case, the speech-language clinician not only needs to establish that the child's language competencies, receptive, expressive, or both, are functioning below age expectations, but also that the child's hearing levels are normal, the child's nonverbal IQ score is within normal limits, there are no obvious gross or fine motor abnormalities, and there are no concerns with the child's social-emotional functioning.

In assessing the presence of language disorders in preschool-age children, these children's cognitive abilities will have to be carefully considered so that tasks selected are within their intellectual reach. Otherwise, we will not know whether the results of our testing say more about the language competencies we believe we are exploring, or are the result of using linguistic or cognitive concepts that were beyond the comprehension of our young clients. It will also be critical to keep in mind how cultural and linguistic variables may impact the assessment process. This issue is incorporated into the procedures recommended in this resource guide, but the reader is referred to Brian Goldstein's book (2000) in this resource guide series for additional assistance.

The assessment/evaluation portion of this section provides information on topics that will aid in determining the presence and scope of a language disorder and is divided into several main subsections:

Subsection I: Preassessment

1. Factors to Consider During Preassessment

2. Suggestions for Observation Protocols

3. Case Histories/Questionnaires

4. Other Sources of Information

5. Determining Risk for Development of Language Disorders

Subsection II: Assessment/Evaluation

1. Special Considerations for SLI

2. Determining the Scope of the Problem

3. Language Assessment Procedures

4. Miscellaneous Procedures and Information

PREASSESSMENT

Prior to initiating any assessment procedures, the clinician should consider gathering information from a number of potential sources, in addition to the clinician's own observations, to determine the child's communication competencies in a number of settings as well as the linguistic demands made on the child during his or her daily routines. Preassessment will also consider issues of the child's family system so that decisions can be made regarding who will participate in the assessment and how that participation will manifest itself. Background information from medical and educational sources may also be relevant to consider before making decisions about the selection of specific assessment tools. This subsection outlines areas that SLPs should consider prior to the formal assessment process.

Observation of Communicative Behaviors During Preassessment

WHO?	All SLPs who provide assessment to preschool-age children. Information can be collected from classroom teachers, family members, and so on.
WHAT?	Gathering background information concerning the child's language competencies in different communication contexts as well as the demands for communication in those contexts.
WHY?	To assist in determining the focus and scope of the assessment test battery.
HOW?	Determine which communicative behaviors are consistently, inconsistently, or never observed through careful observation.
WHERE?	Make observations in any setting where the child spends considerable time and where communication is needed, for example, day care, home, grandparent's home.

Here are some steps for a speech-language pathologist to follow to put together a comprehensive picture of the communicative competencies that a young child typically demonstrates in a variety of communication contexts. These data will be helpful in making decisions regarding whether or not a more in-depth evaluation is necessary and, if so, what the focus of that evaluation should be.

❖ Note that for most of these questions it would be helpful for the clinician's informant to indicate whether the behaviors observed are *consistently observed, inconsistently observed,* or *rarely observed* and if there are specific contexts more likely to elicit these behaviors.

❖ This information may bear a direct connection with eventual targets selected if therapy is deemed appropriate.

  • We assume that behaviors *consistently observed* are within the child's typical repertoire of behaviors (mastered competencies) and will probably not be targeted within treatment.

    – Sometimes these behaviors can be used as the basis, models, or analogies for behaviors to be learned.

    – Example: Child consistently uses a reaching gesture to signal a desired object. Use this as a basis to show that the gesture plus an appropriate word will increase success, especially with new children and adults.

  • Behaviors present but *inconsistently observed* are probably emerging behaviors that the child is working to finesse and represent appropriate targets for treatment.

    – When targeted, these behaviors are probably the easiest for the child to learn.

    – The child has partial knowledge of them.

    – The child may need additional exposure and practice to learn how to generalize their use to additional, similar contexts.

- Example: Child verbalizes requests for action and objects, but not requests for information. Teach: "Go school?"

- Behaviors that are *rarely or never observed* may be too challenging at present for the child because the prerequisite behaviors are not yet in place.

  - These may require the clinician to do a careful task analysis to determine the component parts of the task.

  - Prerequisite skills may need to be addressed prior to the target itself.

  - Example: If the child shows no evidence of a request function, the clinician may need to target use of a gesture or a combination of gesture and vocalization first, then couple it with indication of an object or a person in response to a "Where's X?" question.

❖ *Note:* The main question being asked is: What are the communication demands placed on the child and to what extent can she or he meet those demands?

❖ See the suggested resources on the following pages for additional ideas of observational protocols that can be utilized during preassessment. These protocols largely focus on a young child's pragmatic abilities across a number of settings.

Suggested Case History Forms and Questionnaires

WHO?   SLPs attempting to collect comprehensive background information about how the child uses language.

WHAT?   Formats for collecting this relevant information; suggestions about what to ask when interviewing informants.

WHY?   We want as much information as possible to determine whether a formal evaluation is needed and, if so, to pinpoint possible trouble spots.

WHEN?   These questionnaires and case history formats can be completed as part of a preassessment battery to determine appropriateness of a formal evaluation, or at the same time that standardized tests and nonstandardized probes are administered.

HOW?   See protocols from Bedrosian (1985), Gallagher (1983), and Tomblin, Ellis Weismer, and Weiss (1996) that follow.

Each of these three suggested protocols or sets of protocols in the case of Tomblin et al. (1996) has the potential to provide a clinician with useful information about the extent to which the preschool-age child is able to meet the communication demands placed on him or her either in the classroom or in a home setting. Bedrosian's (1985) checklist, presented in Figure 2–1, specifically focuses on the child's discourse competencies. Titled *A Molar Analysis*, Bedrosian's interest is in delineating both the quality and the quantity (relative frequency) of the child's topic management skills. The checklist can be completed during online observation of the child in a variety of settings and, with some training, caregivers and teachers can be useful information gatherers with this tool.

Gallagher's (1983) preassessment questionnaire, found in Figure 2–2, represents a comprehensive attempt to gather sufficient background information about the quality of a child's communication repertoire. Completion of this questionnaire should provide the clinician with an overview of the manner in which a child handles communication demands at home and/or preschool with a variety of conversation partners, and in a variety of common contexts. The clinician would also derive a better understanding of the caregiver's perspective of the child's communication problem by carefully probing for answers to some of the questions on this protocol.

Tomblin, Ellis Weismer, and Weiss (1996) developed a set of two questionnaires that could be used by classroom teachers and speech-language clinicians. The first, the "Curricular Competencies Checklist," presented in Figure 2–3, was designed to allow for a quick description of a child's ability to meet both the academic and social-communicative demands of the classroom culture with and without accommodations by teaching personnel. The second in the series, also presented in Figure 2–3, is called the "Speech-Language Service Delivery Checklist" and provides the clinician with an opportunity to describe the child's communication problem, the type of treatment programming provided, the child's progress, and the child's conversation skills as observed by the clinician. Although originally designed for use in a specific longitudinal research project, the protocols should have utility when incorporated into the data-gathering process of assessment leading to a full language evaluation.

Following the three protocols, there is a list of questions that can be adapted by SLPs for general data gathering purposes focusing on how children use the language in their repertoires.

Discourse Skills Checklist: A Molar Analysis

Name of Client: _____

Date of interaction: _____

Type of participant interaction: _____

Type of setting: _____

Length of interaction: _____

Instructions: Check the appropriate skill descriptor that follows:

	Yes	No	Sometimes	Not Applicable
I. Topic Initiations				
A. Frequency of client's topic initiations in comparison to the other participant(s): (check one)				
1. None	☐	☐	☐	☐
2. Less than	☐	☐	☐	☐
3. Approximately equal to	☐	☐	☐	☐
4. More than	☐	☐	☐	☐
B. Subject matter of topic initiations:				
1. Able to get attention of listener	☐	☐	☐	☐
2. Repeats old topics on a daily basis	☐	☐	☐	☐
3. Initiates new topics on a daily basis	☐	☐	☐	☐
4. Able to greet others	☐	☐	☐	☐
5. Able to express departures when leaving	☐	☐	☐	☐
6. Able to make introductions	☐	☐	☐	☐
7. Able to initiate needs	☐	☐	☐	☐
8. Able to initiate questions:	☐	☐	☐	☐
a. Requests for information	☐	☐	☐	☐
b. Requests for repetition or clarification	☐	☐	☐	☐
c. Requests for action	☐	☐	☐	☐
d. Requests for permission	☐	☐	☐	☐
9. Talks mostly about self	☐	☐	☐	☐
10. Talks about the other, as well as self	☐	☐	☐	☐
11. Talks about referents in the past	☐	☐	☐	☐
12. Talks about referents in the future	☐	☐	☐	☐
13. Talks about referents in the present	☐	☐	☐	☐
14. Talks about fantasy-related referents	☐	☐	☐	☐
15. Calls people names	☐	☐	☐	☐
16. Uses noise or sound-word play in appropriate situations	☐	☐	☐	☐

Figure 2–1. Bedrosian's (1985) Discourse Skills Checklist: A Molar Analysis

	Yes	No	Sometimes	Not Applicable

II. Maintaining Topics

   A. Able to keep a topic going:

	Yes	No	Sometimes	Not Applicable
1. Responds to questions	☐	☐	☐	☐
2. Acknowledges topic (e.g., "Uh-huh")	☐	☐	☐	☐
3. Offers new information that is related	☐	☐	☐	☐
4. Requests more information about a topic	☐	☐	☐	☐
5. Able to ask requests for repetition or clarification if message is not clear	☐	☐	☐	☐
6. Able to repeat or answer questions about what another has talked about	☐	☐	☐	☐
7. Agrees with others	☐	☐	☐	☐
8. Disagrees with others	☐	☐	☐	☐

   B. Not able to keep a topic going:

	Yes	No	Sometimes	Not Applicable
1. Intentionally evades or ignores a question	☐	☐	☐	☐
2. Initiates a topic immediately following a topic initiation by a prior speaker	☐	☐	☐	☐
3. Engages in monologues when in a group	☐	☐	☐	☐

III. Use of Eye Contact

	Yes	No	Sometimes	Not Applicable
A. Able to use eye contact to designate a listener in a group when initiating a topic	☐	☐	☐	☐
B. Uses eye contact while listening	☐	☐	☐	☐

IV. Turn-taking

	Yes	No	Sometimes	Not Applicable
A. Is easily interrupted	☐	☐	☐	☐
B. Interrupts others	☐	☐	☐	☐
C. Answers questions for others	☐	☐	☐	☐
D. Has long speaking turns	☐	☐	☐	☐
E. Designates turns for others in a group	☐	☐	☐	☐
F. Sensitive to listener cues (e.g., can tell if listener is interested or bored)	☐	☐	☐	☐
G. Excuses self when interrupting	☐	☐	☐	☐

V. Politeness

	Yes	No	Sometimes	Not Applicable
A. Able to make indirect requests	☐	☐	☐	☐
B. Uses commands	☐	☐	☐	☐
C. Uses politeness markers of "Please," "Thank you," "Excuse me"	☐	☐	☐	☐

VI. Observation of Nonverbal Behaviors

	Yes	No	Sometimes	Not Applicable
A. Stands or sits too close to people when talking	☐	☐	☐	☐
B. Stands or sits too far away from people when talking	☐	☐	☐	☐
C. Stands or sits at appropriate social distances when talking	☐	☐	☐	☐
D. Uses nonverbal head nods to acknowledge	☐	☐	☐	☐
E. Uses nonverbal means of getting attention to initiate a topic (e.g., taps on shoulder, points)	☐	☐	☐	☐

Preassessment Questionnaire

Tanya M. Gallagher

Developmental Language Programs
Communicative Disorders Clinic
The University of Michigan

(All information in this questionnaire will be considered confidential)

Child's Name _____ Birthdate _____

Address _____ Sex _____

Name of person filling out questionnaire _____

Relationship to child _____

List children and adults who live in child's home other than the parents:

Name _____ Age _____ Relationship _____

Name _____ Age _____ Relationship _____

Name _____ Age _____ Relationship _____

Name _____ Age _____ Relationship _____

Who recommended that the child's communicative behavior be assessed?

Name _____ Relationship to child _____

How did the above person describe the child's communicative difficulties? _____

_____

_____

_____

Have others commented upon the child's communicative difficulties? If so, what were these comments? _____

_____

_____

_____

Have you consulted other professionals regarding the child's communicative difficulties? _____

Whom _____

What were the recommendations? _____

_____

What things have you tried to change the child's communicative behavior? Describe: _____

_____

_____

Describe the child's communicative behavior as completely as possible: _____

_____

_____

_____

_____

_____

_____

Figure 2–2. A Preassessment Questionnaire Developed by Gallagher (1983)

Does the child's communicative behavior change relative to that description when he talks with:

1. A friend? Name _____ Age _____ What changes do you observe?
_____
_____

2. A younger sibling? Name _____ Age _____ What changes do you observe?
_____

3. An older sibling? Name _____ Age _____ What changes do you observe?
_____

4. A teacher (or someone in authority)? What changes do you observe? _____
_____
_____

5. Mother? What changes do you observe? _____
_____
_____

6. Father? What changes do you observe? _____
_____
_____

7. Familiar adult (neighbor, grandparent, etc.)? What changes do you observe? _____
_____
_____

8. Unfamiliar adult (sales persons, etc.)? What changes do you observe? _____
_____
_____

9. Small group? What changes do you observe? _____
_____
_____

Does the child's communicative behavior change relative to your original description when he talks about:

1. Things he has done? How? _____
_____
_____

2. Things he will do? How? _____
_____
_____

3. Things he is doing? How? _____
_____
_____

4. Things someone else is doing? How? _____
_____
_____

(continued)

Figure 2–2. *(continued)*

5. Familiar toys or activities? How? _____
_____
_____

6. Unfamiliar toys or activities? How? _____
_____
_____

7. What are your child's favorite playthings? _____
_____
_____

8. What activities does your child enjoy participating in? _____
_____
_____

9. Describe how your child plays with his favorite playmates: _____
_____
_____

Of the following, recommend what would probably be the child's best communicative situation:
Who _____
When (time of day) _____
Place _____
Activities _____
Objects _____
Other _____

Relative to the following, recommend what would probably be the child's most frequent communicative situation:
Who _____
When (time of day) _____
Place _____
Activities _____
Objects _____
Other _____

Curricular Competencies Checklist
Child Language Research Center

Student's Name: _____   Date: _____

Teacher's Name: _____

1. Please rate this student in terms of how well he or she does in tasks focusing on each of the following academic competency areas. Circle the number that best reflects your opinion. Consider the student's performance relative to grade-level expectation.

	Significantly Below	Somewhat Below	At Grade Level	Somewhat Above	Significantly Above
Speaking	1	2	3	4	5
Listening	1	2	3	4	5
Reading	1	2	3	4	5
Writing	1	2	3	4	5
Math	1	2	3	4	5

2. To what degree is this student meeting the following expectations of the classroom curriculum?

	Significantly Below	Somewhat Below	At Grade Level	Somewhat Above	Significantly Above
Academic	1	2	3	4	5
Social	1	2	3	4	5

3. Please rate this student's potential for progress within this school year. Circle the number that best reflects your opinion.

(1)	(2)	(3)	(4)	(5)
Significantly (Below Expectations)	Somewhat	Expected Rate	Somewhat	Significantly (Above Expectations)

4. In many classrooms, students are asked to learn in different contexts. To what degree is this student meeting the expectations of the following instructional settings?

	Significantly Below	Somewhat Below	At Grade Level	Somewhat Above	Significantly Above
Teacher–Student (whole class)	1	2	3	4	5
Teacher–Student (small group)	1	2	3	4	5
Student & student	1	2	3	4	5
Student alone	1	2	3	4	5

5. To facilitate this student's success in the classroom, is it necessary for you to adapt your teaching methods in any way?

Yes   No

If yes, what percentage of time do you adapt your teaching methods? _____

Figure 2–3. The Curricular Competencies Checklist Developed by Tomblin et al. (1996)

(continued)

Figure 2–3. *(continued)*

6. Is this student able to participate in conversations where partners share equally in the responsibilities of listening and communicating?

Yes	No

7. Does this student communicate in conversations in a manner that is similar to his or her same-age peers?

Yes	No

8. Please describe this student's conversational skills using the three point scale.

This student:

	Never	Sometimes	Very Often
Talks too much	0	1	2
Talks too little	0	1	2
Interrupts others who are talking	0	1	2
Talks at the same time others are talking	0	1	2
Introduces appropriate topics of conversation	0	1	2
Maintains the topic of conversation	0	1	2
Answers conversational questions appropriately	0	1	2
Demonstrates different conversational behaviors with peers versus adults	0	1	2

9. Is this student currently receiving speech/language therapy?

Yes	No

Speech-Language Service Delivery Checklist
Child Language Research Center

Student's Name: _____   Date: _____

Speech-Language Pathologist's Name: _____

1. How long has this student been receiving speech-language services on your caseload?

2. To the best of your knowledge, how long has this student been receiving speech-language services from any speech-language clinician?

3. At this time, is this student receiving services for any other the following? (Please check all that apply)

Learning disability _____

Cognitive disability _____

Emotional/behavioral disability _____

Visual impairment _____

Physical/motor involvement _____

Hearing impairment _____

Others? _____ _____

4. If direct services are being provided, indicate the *frequency* and *length* of speech/language intervention sessions this student is receiving.

5. What type of service delivery model is currently used with this student? Please circle the option(s) that best describes the intervention model and then indicate the approximate amount of time spent in each option.

Treatment Type	Amount of Time
Consultation only (no direct service)	_____
Classroom collaboration (co-teaching)	_____
Contextually-based (in the classroom but not co-teaching)	_____
Pull-out, individual	_____
Pull-out, small group	_____
Parent training	_____
Normal language peer models	_____
Other _____	_____

6. What type of treatment goal(s) have you designated for this student? Please check all that apply.

Oral Language	_____	Pragmatics	_____
Phonology/Articulation	_____	Voice	_____
Fluency	_____	Reading	_____
Written Language	_____	Others: _____	

Figure 2–3. Speech-Language Service Delivery Checklist Developed by Tomblin et al. (1996)

(continued)

Figure 2–3. *(continued)*

7. If any of your treatment goals include *language*, please describe the type of treatment approach(es) that you are using for these goals. Check all that apply. If none apply, please add more appropriate descriptions under "Others."

Whole language	_____
Direct instruction (Drill/practice/imitation)	_____
Learning strategies (Study skills, memory aids, organizational skills)	_____
Curriculum-based	_____
Incidental teaching/Milieu therapy	_____
Computer-assisted instruction	_____
Reading-based approach (e.g., Communicative Reading Strategies by Janet Norris)	_____
Language experience/Interactive approach (Modeling during activities with opportunities to respond)	_____

Others: _____

8. How would you rate this child's progress during the time he/she has been on your caseload? Circle the number that most accurately reflects where you believe this student falls on a continuum of "expected rate of progress."

(1)	(2)	(3)	(4)	(5)
Significantly (Below Expectations)	Somewhat	Expected Rate	Somewhat	Significantly (Above Expectations)

9. To what do you attribute this student's rate of progress in treatment? Check all that apply.

Cognitive Abilities	_____	Motivation	_____
Effectiveness of Treatment Program	_____	Maturity	_____

Others? _____

10. Is this student able to participate in conversations where partners share equally in the responsibilities of listening and communicating?

Yes   No

11. Does this student communicate in conversations in a manner that is similiar to his or her same-age peers?

Yes   No

12. Please describe this student's conversational skills using the three point scale. This student:

	Never	Sometimes	Always
Talks too much	0	1	2
Talks too little	0	1	2
Interrupts others who are talking	0	1	2
Talks at the same time others are talking	0	1	2
Initiates conversations	0	1	2
Maintains topics for more than one turn	0	1	2
Answers conversational questions appropriately	0	1	2
Demonstrates different conversational behaviors with peers versus adults	0	1	2

Clinical Insight

For some clinical cases, it may make sense to use more than one observational protocol or questionnaire so do not view these as mutually exclusive. SLPs should not hesitate to be creative and add or eliminate questions to these preexisting protocols to make each one a better fit for a particular client or family. None of these are standardized instruments so making some changes to the protocol will not alter the instrument's statistical validity as an information-gathering device. Also note that data can be gathered by observation only, from caregiver report, by setting up a contrived situation creating the opportunity for a communication behavior to be produced, or by a combination of these methods.

Suggestions for Gathering Information about Young Children's Language Competencies
(Collecting Information from a Variety of Informants Familiar with the Child)

❖ Who spends the most time with the child during the day?

❖ Does the child attend a day care or preschool program?

❖ If so, how long has the child attended this program?

❖ Is the child well integrated into the daily activities of the preschool or day care setting? That is, is the child familiar with the routine and able to participate when asked to join in?

❖ Is the child considered to be a "popular" child by his or her peers? By the teacher?

❖ Does the child both initiate conversations with other children in the classroom and respond to the conversational "bids" (Fey, 1986) made by classmates? With teachers?

❖ Does the child ask for clarification from a peer or the teacher if directions are unclear?

❖ Does the child recognize when the listener is confused and needs clarification?

❖ Does the child have a *variety* of strategies for providing clarification, for example, imitation, elaboration, and word substitution, if clarification is needed by a conversation partner?

❖ Does the child appear able to follow the rules of the general classroom routine, such as joining in group activities when requested, depositing personal belongings in his or her own locker?

❖ Is the child able to take a turn in talking? During games? Other classroom activities?

❖ Is the child a risk taker in terms of trying activities that are somewhat challenging whether these be language-based or academic skill-based or motor skill-based?

❖ When the child is frustrated, does he or she use words or gestures in an attempt to explain feelings and ask for assistance or does the child resort to disruptive acting out behaviors?

❖ What sorts of specific directions is the child expected to be able to follow within the confines of daily classroom (or at-home) activities?

❖ What sorts of behavior management techniques are utilized in the classroom (or at home)?

❖ Is the child generally included in the conversations of other children?

❖ Does the child appear to avoid situations where talking will be a requirement?

❖ Does the child demonstrate any awareness of difficulty communicating?

SUMMARY

A. Communication behaviors consistently observed:

B. Communication behaviors inconsistently observed:

C. Communication behaviors rarely/never observed:

D. Contexts that increase likelihood of appropriate communication skills, for example,

- What types of support, provided by a caregiver, teacher, or other professional, are likely to facilitate the child's ability to meet the communication demands presented?

- In what physical settings is the child more likely to succeed, for example, in small groups of children, when working one-on-one with the classroom teacher, at home, and so on?

- What types of materials tend to increase the likelihood that the child will succeed with communication tasks, for example, use of objects rather than pictures, use of photographs to support the child's relating of stories?

Other Sources of Information

> **WHO?** All SLPs who provide assessment services to preschool-age children.
>
> **WHAT?** Collection of background information regarding medical, psychological, social, and communicative abilities from professional sources.
>
> **WHY?** This information assists in determining the need for evaluation as well as the focus and scope of that evaluation.
>
> **HOW?** Once appropriate, legal releases are obtained, information can be gathered directly from the source or via written documentation.

Ideally, information from these sources should be collected prior to the planning of the assessment/evaluation session(s) to allow you time to digest the information and use it in evaluation planning. In reality, it often arrives after the evaluation. Most of the time, families are forthcoming in their willingness to facilitate the conveyance of this information to you, but, in some instances, the clinician may meet with resistance from family members.

> **Clinical Insight**
>
> In some instances, especially when parents or another primary caregiver ask you to provide them with a second opinion, you may not be given permission to obtain reports of the findings of other professionals. The family may be concerned that seeing these other reports will bias your decision making.

In most situations you will have to gain legal permission to request and receive reports from other professionals. Facilities should have these permission forms in place to comply with local and federal regulations. Release forms should be updated annually.

❖ **Pertinent Medical Information**

- If the child is receiving ongoing treatment or being monitored for a chronic ailment, such as allergies, asthma, an oral-facial anomaly, and so on, current reports from the child's physician may yield relevant information. For example, if the child is regularly taking antihistamines for allergies, apparent attention deficits may be drug-related, if sleepiness is a side effect of the medication.

- Is the child currently taking any medications on a daily basis? If so, for what conditions? Inquire about any side effects the child may habitually experience for daily medications.

- Is there a history of general concern regarding growth and development? Is this a child who showed, or still shows, signs of "failure to thrive"?

- Have referrals been made by the family or others connected with the family to other professionals to provide specific treatment, either for the child or the family?

- social workers
- psychologists/family therapists
- occupational therapists
- visiting nurses or home-based educators

- Is there relevant family, medical, or social history that may impact this child's health and well-being?
  - History of abuse?
  - History of neglect?
  - History of extended illness or hospitalization of the primary caregiver(s)?

❖ **Pertinent Psychological Information**

- Has the child been evaluated by a psychologist or psychiatrist due to concerns about specific aberrant child behaviors?
  - Suspicion of obsessive/compulsive disorder; general mental health?
  - Have there been episodes of depression or anxiety?

- Has the child received any drug treatment or counseling for a psychological disorder?

- Is the child presently on medication or receiving counseling for such a problem?

- Has the child been tested to evaluate his or her ability to learn and to make recommendations for the best learning environments for the child?

- If the child has received educational testing, were the tests selected chosen for their nonbiased characteristics?
  - That is, Performance Scale IQ tests attempt to reduce or eliminate the language load from the child's responses.
  - This is critical in the testing of children where language problems are known or suspected.
  - If inappropriate testing has been completed, arranging appropriate testing may be necessary.

❖ **Pertinent Social Information**

- Information may potentially be collected from the child's primary caregiver(s), other family members including siblings and members of the extended family, his or her classroom teacher if the child attends school, or from social workers if one has been involved with the child's family.

- Information should focus on the child's development of social-emotional or self-help skills. Several examples of these skills follow:
  - Is the child feeding himself/herself?
  - Is the child dressing himself/herself?
  - Is the child toilet trained during the day? At night?
  - Does the child easily form friendships with same-age peers?
  - How does the child deal with conflicts with other children? With caregivers?

❖ Pertinent Communication Information

- This information can be gleaned from the SLP's observations of the child's communication environments as well as from the reports of primary and secondary caregivers.

- What communication demands or expectations are placed on the child during his/her activities of daily living? Most of these questions have also been included in the questionnaires already presented.

- To what degree is the child able to meet those demands or expectations?

- To what degree is the child apparently aware of the communication expectations and demands in his or her environment?

- In situations where the child cannot meet those demands or expectations, how does the child respond or deal with these situations?
  - Mostly linguistically?
  - Mostly nonlinguistically?
  - By using a combination of linguistic and nonlinguistic means?

- Are there contexts in which the child is a more successful communicator?

- Are there contexts in which the child is a less successful communicator?

Risk Factors for Developing a Language Disorder

WHO?	SLPs involved in the diagnosis and treatment of young children.
WHAT?	Children may exhibit risk factors, or red flags that increase the likelihood that they will develop a language disorder.
WHY?	Although a child may still function within the normal range of language skill expectation, early intervention may be called for to diminish the effect of a potential problem or eliminate its occurrence.
HOW?	Usually through provision of treatment in the home environment by caregivers, SLPs, or trained home care providers or monitoring by SLPs for change.
WHEN?	Early intervention is viewed as best practice for treating a child exhibiting risk factors for developing language disorders.

Many researchers believe that the benefit of early intervention services has been clearly demonstrated (Ramey & Ramey, 1998) and, therefore, efforts focusing on identification of a potential language problem as early as possible are warranted. Where do we look and who can assist us?

❖ Because reliable and valid instruments for the diagnosis of language disorders in very young children are few and far between, we cannot always rely on standardized testing to pinpoint potential problems in young children.

❖ Concern expressed by primary caregivers and/or extended family members that the child is not progressing normally should be viewed seriously by the clinician.

❖ Concern expressed by day care providers that the child is not progressing at the same rate as other children the same age in language acquisition or social-emotional development.

❖ The presence of one or more risk factors for the normal development of language.

• Biological risk factors

  – Birth history including pre-, peri-, postnatal trauma

  – Genetic history that is often compatible with development of a language disorder, for example, presence of a syndrome such as "Fragile X," Down syndrome

  – Presence of a significant sensorineural hearing loss detected shortly after birth

  – History of recurrent middle ear infections and concomitant hearing loss

• Familial risk factors

  – Very young parents with limited support network

  – Caregivers with a history of drug and alcohol abuse

  – Caregivers with a history of child neglect and/or abuse

- Other environmental risk factors

  - Exposure to drugs in utero, including alcohol (fetal alcohol syndrome, fetal alcohol effect)

  - Inconsistent health care, for example, children may not have a consistent primary health care provider or manager; health services are provided in the emergency room

  - Insufficient funds available for adequate housing, food, clothing

  - Inadequate exposure to language models

  - Inadequate exposure to educational stimuli such as printed materials

- Communicative/Behavioral risk factors

  - Slow development of expressive and receptive vocabulary. This topic was considered in more detail regarding "late talkers" in Section 1. Note that several groups of investigators believe that delayed acquisition of first words and late acquisition of word combinations predict SLI for between 25% and 50% of children (Leonard, 1998). Note as well the high rate of "recovery" to normal language parameters.

  - Evidence of inability or unwillingness to attend to pertinent auditory input.

  - Evidence of inability or unwillingness to produce rudimentary, non-verbal or verbal communicative attempts.

  - Evidence of inability or unwillingness to communicatively engage children or adults in meaningful ways.

  - Evidence of rigidity in the child's activities, for example, difficulty changing from one activity to another or difficulty with having others initiate activities with the child.

  - Catastrophic responses, for example, tantruming when exposed to minimal environmental changes.

  - Child "acts out," perhaps out of the frustration of not being able to communicate.

Clinical Insight

Ramey and Ramey (1998) identified what they called six "developmental priming mechanisms," (p. 115) among them: encouragement for environmental exploration, sufficient language and symbolic communication stimulation, opportunities to rehearse and expand new skills, and availability for mentoring in basic cognitive and social skills, strongly associated with positive developmental outcomes.

ASSESSMENT/EVALUATION

Special Considerations for Evaluating SLI

WHO?	All SLPs who suspect that the language disorder they are evaluating would be better described as Specific Language Impairment (SLI). However, specific testing, for example, hearing and cognitive abilities, may be more appropriately evaluated by another professional with specialized training.
WHAT?	Assessment of the specific factors that discriminate SLI.
WHY?	A diagnosis of SLI may carry with it different implications for treatment than for the child without SLI.
HOW?	Complete a comprehensive history as suggested below.
LITERATURE RESOURCES	Leonard (1998), Plante (1996), and Stark and Tallal (1981).

Areas of evaluation follow that should be explored in order to delineate the presence of SLI. SLPs may want to view this as a checklist for deciding on the questions to be answered as part of the child's evaluation.

❖ **Hearing Ability:** Is the child's hearing adequate for language learning?

- Any child with a suspected language disorder should always receive hearing testing.

- Should be tested by means of pure-tone threshold testing, tympanometry/acoustic reflexes, and speech discrimination testing to rule out significant hearing loss.

- Hearing thresholds should be no higher than 20 dB HL.

- Tympanograms should demonstrate normal peak pressures.

- Speech reception thresholds should be no greater than 20 dB HL.

- Make sure that you have the results of the hearing testing prior to beginning formal assessment.

- Results allow you to make any necessary accommodations in your test setting or in the selection of where or how you do the assessment.

- Is the child's present hearing acuity sufficient to support language learning through the auditory system and, if not, is referral for hearing augmentation needed?

- Remember to incorporate this information into recommendations for family-child communicative interactions as well as those in any preschool classroom environments.

❖ **Cognitive Ability:** Is the child's intellectual functioning commensurate with the child's language abilities?

- Nonverbal IQ measures derived from *Performance Scale* tests are supposed to minimally tap into the child's verbal skills so as not to bias test results.

- Ideally, psychologists with specialized training in testing children with special needs are utilized to select, administer, and interpret these tests.

- Several tests frequently used for this purpose are:

  - *Wechsler Intelligence Scale for Children-Revised (WISC-R)* (Wechsler, 1974)

  - *Wechsler Preschool and Primary Scale of Intelligence-Revised (WPPSI-R)* (Wechsler, 1989)

  - *Columbia Mental Maturity Scale (CMMS)* (Burgemeister, Blum, & Lorge, 1972)

  - *Test of Nonverbal Intelligence (TONI)* (Brown, Sherbenou, & Johnson, 1982)

  - *Kaufman Assessment Battery for Children (KABC)* (Kaufman & Kaufman, 1983)

- Be aware that there is some controversy regarding the appropriate IQ cut-off for consideration of SLI. This controversy stems from consideration of 85 (High SLIs) or 70 (Low SLIs), according to Tomblin (1997). Fey, Long, and Cleave (1994) also discuss this issue at length.

❖ **Motor Functioning:** Are the child's motor skills commensurate with what is necessary to explore the child's world, perform self-help activities, and communicate with gestures, with speech, or with written symbols?

- Observe directly or learn from an informant about the adequacy of the child's gross or large muscle motor skills when the child is at play, for example, walking, running, jumping, hopping, and skipping.

- Observe directly or learn from an informant about the adequacy of the child's fine or small muscle motor skills when the child is engaged in classroom activities, for example, holding and using crayons and other drawing implements; using "child" scissors; copying letters, numbers, shapes; feeding self; dressing and undressing self (outer wear at school and additional articles of clothes at home); and so on.

- Is the child able to use a conventional set of gestures for communicative purposes, for example, pointing, showing, giving, for requesting?

- Is the child's speech intelligible enough to be communicative? *Note:* Some investigators use the symptomatology of developmental apraxia of speech, a disorder that renders children highly unintelligible, as an exclusionary factor for SLI. Others do not view this as reason to exclude the diagnosis of SLI.

  - See definitions of developmental apraxia of speech in the following resources: Crary (1993); Hall, Jordan, and Robin (1993); Velleman and Strand (1994).

- Is the child demonstrating any difficulties with production of volitional oral motor movements including swallowing? Performance of an oral mechanism exam (see Hall's section in Tomblin, Morris, & Spriestersbach, 1999) will help the clinician delineate the presence and extent of the problem.

❖ **Social-Emotional Functioning:** Are there significant concerns about the child's social development that would suggest the presence of a diagnosis of autism?

- Does the child separate easily from the primary caregiver to work with an unfamiliar but friendly adult (a situation that often occurs in the early stages of treatment)?

- Does the child demonstrate difficulty, perhaps manifested as anxiety or fear, in transitioning from one activity to another, that is, rigidity?

- Does the child tend to perseverate in one activity until moved to another activity by an adult or another, older child?

- Does the child exhibit compulsivity or impulsivity in play behaviors or when asked to complete a task?

- Do the primary caregiver(s), teachers, or others express concerns about the child's personality development?

- Does the child attempt to communicate verbally or nonverbally with other children or tend to ignore them?

- Does the child play appropriately with other children who are the same age? We know that children's play behaviors progressively develop from nontangential, to parallel, to cooperative play during the preschool years.

- Use of a test instrument like the *Child Behavior Checklist (CBCL)* (Achenbach, 1991) is a tool often used by psychologists and others to identify children, ages 4 through 18, who may have social adjustment problems necessitating intervention.

  – Test forms are questionnaires.

  – There are separate forms for classroom teachers and parents to complete.

  – Normative data allow examiners to compare their client's performance with the performance of children who have been referred for psychological or psychiatric care.

- One of the chief disorders or syndromes to rule out is autism, a phenomenon that may be more correctly viewed as a spectrum of related types of communication problems, thus the term "Autism Spectrum Disorder" (Prelock, 1999).

  – The origins are not fully understood and may be neurochemical or otherwise neurological in nature.

  – Some practitioners use the term *pervasive developmental disorder* interchangeably with autism, but this is not a very descriptive or helpful term.

  – There is little agreement on the composite of characteristics that must be present to warrant a diagnosis of autism.

  – Children with autism often have delayed language onset, may have no oral/expressive language, produce few communicative attempts, and/or demonstrate bizarre or deviant language patterns, that is, patterns not observed in normally developing children.

  – It is not uncommon for the primary caregiver of a child with autism to report that the child no longer uses the language she or he once used, for example, smaller vocabulary, incomplete sentences, or no longer speaks at all.

– It is also not uncommon for the caregiver to report that the young child, although not using much language to communicate, has shown evidence of **hyperlexia**, that is, early reading ability.

– Typically, hyperlexia amounts to the child being able to make the symbol-sound connections but being unable to derive meaning from them. That is, it is a noncommunicative skill.

– A good resource for further information about autism spectrum disorders is the Web site for the Center for the Study of Autism; the address is http://www.autism.org.

Determining the Scope of the Problem

WHO? All SLPs interested in carefully delineating the language difficulties exhibited by preschool-age children.

WHAT? Though standardized tests provide some critical information concerning the severity of the problem, it will likely take the inclusion of nonstandardized probes to fully answer this question.

WHY? This combination of information is crucial for diagnosis, treatment planning, and providing some prognostic information.

HOW? By utilizing nonstandardized probes to shore up the deficits of the standardized testing or carefully assembling a comprehensive test battery or both.

LITERATURE RESOURCES See Leonard, Prutting, Perozzi, and Berkeley (1978); Lund and Duchan (1993); Weiss, Tomblin, and Robin (1999).

In addition to determining whether a problem exists, the assessment phase of the clinical process also serves to describe the *scope* of the problem, should a problem exist. Standardized tests alone cannot be expected to fulfill this need; that is not their primary purpose. Results of standardized tests must be augmented by the use of nonstandardized probes that are often designed by clinicians to meet the particular needs of the clinician by answering the particular questions necessary to determine where treatment should begin. That can mean:

❖ Does the problem exist in both language comprehension and production?

- For the child with SLI this may be particularly important because research has shown that the child with problems in the area of expressive language only has a better prognosis for catching up with age-expected levels of performance than does the child who demonstrates difficulties with both language comprehension and expression (Beitchman, 1985; Bishop & Edmundson, 1987).

- SLPs will want to be sure to put together test batteries that evaluate both the receptive and expressive natures of all language components, for example, vocabulary or syntax, that may be in question.

- Some of the standardized tests that serve to evaluate preschool-age children, such as the *Preschool Language Scale-3 (PLS-3)* (Zimmerman, Steiner, & Pond, 1992) and the *Test of Language Development-3P (TOLD-3P)* (Newcomer & Hammill, 1997) are designed to evaluate both language comprehension and production.

- Other tests focus exclusively on one domain or the other, such as the *Test of Auditory Comprehension for Language-3 (TACL-3)* (Carrow-Woolfolk, 1999) and the *Peabody Picture Vocabulary Test-III (PPVT-III)* (Dunn & Dunn, 1997) for comprehension.

- For young children who appear to be delayed in the beginning stages of language learning, assessment of vocabulary development, use of gestures, and early word combinations can be easily evaluated in a standardized manner by utilizing parent report in a checklist format.

– *The MacArthur Communicative Development Inventory* (Fenson, Dale, Reznick, Thal, Bates, Hartung, Pethick, & Reilly, 1993)

– *The Language Development Survey* (Rescorla, 1989)

❖ How would we characterize the severity of the problem? Is the problem one that demonstrates itself to be both *statistically significant* (child's scores place him or her more than 1.5–2 standard deviations below the mean) and *clinically significant* (child's performance relates to an inability to successfully communicate with others, especially those unfamiliar with the child's language patterns)?

❖ Does the difficulty the child experiences with a particular language form, structure, or function extend to all examples, or almost all examples, of that form, structure, or function or does the child demonstrate partial learning of the language aspect?

- Standardized tests by nature cannot evaluate all examples of all language aspects.

- Their "representative sampling" of items that tap into the child's knowledge of different question forms, for example, may be limited to just a few question types.

- A standardized test may utilize particular items that, because of the vocabulary used or *task* used, are failed by the child whereas other items with different vocabulary and a different task might be responded to with ease.

- The danger of *not* performing nonstandardized probes is that clinicians may end up targeting forms or functions that are already within the child's repertoire and wasting valuable treatment time.

- Nonstandardized probes are developed to allow the clinician to probe more deeply into the problem and determine its scope.

- Another benefit of the nonstandardized probe is that it often lends itself to a greater degree of naturalness in testing: there is less decontextualized language use.

- Often, nonstandardized probes are performed as part of diagnostic therapy and not at the time of the initial evaluation because their development is typically based on the results of a standardized test.

- In order to develop a nonstandardized probe, you will need to know the available tasks at your disposal for assessing receptive and expressive language.

- For some suggestions for how tasks for evaluating receptive and expressive competencies differ in degree of difficulty, see Figure 2–4: "Tasks typically used to assess receptive and expressive language abilities depicted on a continuum representing most to least contextual support" (from Weiss, Tomblin, & Robin, 1999, p. 142).

- You will probably want to alternate the tasks used from those used on the standardized test, for example, if picture identification was used on the test, an "acting out" task with three-dimensional stimuli could be developed.

- An example of how to develop your own nonstandardized probe to assist you in determining the scope of the problem follows.

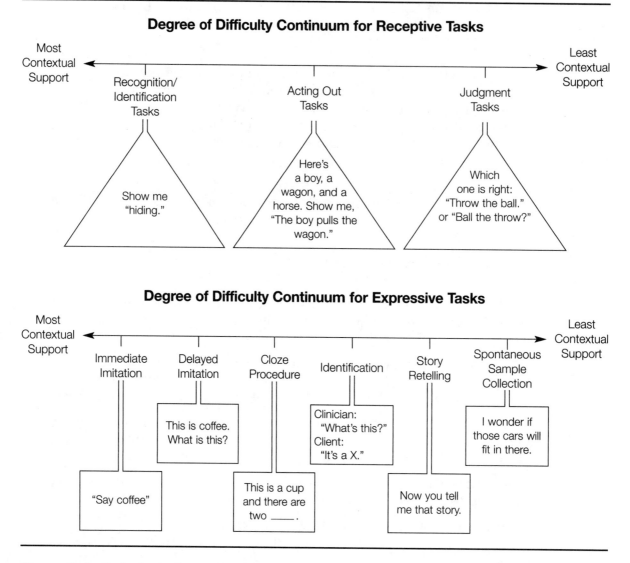

Figure 2–4. Tasks typically used to assess receptive and expressive language abilities depicted on a continuum representing most to least contextual support (From "Language Disorders," by A. Weiss, J. Tomblin, and D. Robin, 1999, p. 142. In J. Tomblin, H. Morris, and D. Spriestersbach [Eds.], *Diagnosis in Speech-Language Pathology*. San Diego, CA: Singular Publishing Group. Copyright 1999 Singluar Publishing Group. Reprinted with permission.)

Development of Nonstandardized Probes

WHO?   SLPs who want to fine-tune their evaluations of children's language abilities.

WHAT? Create a probe to fit the particular language competence/skill/target you need to examine in more depth.

WHY?   Reliance on standardized testing can underestimate or overestimate a child's abilities and thus make goal-setting more problematic.

WHEN? Utilize the results of standardized testing as a key for the focus of the follow-up probes.

HOW?   Follow the procedure subsequently outlined by substituting information about your client's particular needs and language performance on standardized measures.

LITERATURE RESOURCE Leonard et al., 1978.

Here are the steps you can follow to develop a nonstandardized probe that will be useful as part of your evaluation for a preschool-age client.

Clinical Insight

When we talk about nonstandardized probe development and application, we may be talking about using the probes during the evaluation itself or as an activity integral to diagnostic therapy. That is, we do not always have the time to administer a nonstandardized probe at the time of the evaluation proper, let alone develop a nonstandardized probe on line. Of course, if you know ahead of time that the child has a difficult time understanding and producing question forms, you can develop the probe ad hoc and use it at the time of the evaluation. Many times, however, we cannot decide the focus of our nonstandardized probes until we have completed appropriate standardized testing.

❖ Select the language competency you want to test more fully using one or more of the following criteria:
  • the test item was one that should have been within the child's repertoire as per the client's chronological age or developmental age,
  • you suspect that the item(s) on the test were in some way biased against the child's best performance (e.g., words were unfamiliar to the child due to developmental or cultural differences),
  • few items on the test assessed this particular language competence,
  • the items on the test provided insight into the child's receptive ability with this language target but not production, or vice versa.

❖ Select the type of task you want to use to more fully assess the language target or competency.
  • You may want to select a task that is different from the one used on the standardized test to reduce the possibility that it was the task and not the language item being tested that caused the child's difficulty.

❖ Assemble a series of items that will more comprehensively evaluate this language target or competency.

❖ Example: Comprehension of Wh-questions (after Leonard et al., 1978)

- The *Test of Auditory Comprehension of Language-3* (*TACL-3*) (Carrow-Woolfolk, 1999) has two subtests containing items intended to evaluate Wh-question comprehension. In total there are four such questions.

- Given the pervasiveness of Wh-questions in the child's linguistic environment and the importance of their comprehension, a more complete evaluation of a child's Wh-question comprehension is necessary for your client.

- Develop a listing of Wh-questions with several items per Wh-word. Use topics and lexical items within the reference of typical preschool-age children, for example, "Where is the orange?" versus "Where do you usually find a monkey?"

- Use normative data from research studies to guide your selection of items for testing.

   – In the case of Wh-question acquisition, the following sources may prove useful: Parnell, Patterson, and Harding (1984) for comprehension; and Tyack and Ingram (1977) for both comprehension and expression.

- Using Parnell, Patterson, and Harding's (1984) categories in their study of 3-, 4-, 5-, and 6-year-olds, the following nine question types were used:

   – What + be, *What is that?*

   – Which, *Which doggie is fattest?*

   – Where, *Where do you sleep?*

   – Who, *Who drives your car?*

   – Whose, *Whose umbrella is that?*

   – What + do, *What is he doing?*

   – Why, *Why is she crying?*

   – When, *When do you eat breakfast?*

   – What happened, *What happened to the old shoes?*

- At least five examples per question type are used either "naturally" embedded in conversation or by systematically asking the child the questions in a random order with or without the use of supporting materials, as needed.

- For example, for the *Why?* question, use of a baby doll with accompanying muffled sobs may be an appropriate ploy.

- Examine the child's answers for their "functional accuracy" and/or "functional appropriateness" as per Parnell et al. (1984).

- Results of the probe testing will provide the examiner with a better grasp on the scope of the child's abilities or needs in the area of Wh-question comprehension than did standardized testing.

- Decisions about the appropriateness of targeting Wh-questions as a goal can now be made as well as determining the particular Wh-questions that should become objectives in treatment.

Nonstandardized Probe for Wh-Questions

	Functionally Accurate	Functionally Appropriate
What + be, for example, *What is that?*	_____	_____
What is an apple?	_____	_____
What says, "Moo"?	_____	_____
What flies in the sky?	_____	_____
What game do you like to play?	_____	_____
Which, for example, *Which doggie is fattest?*	_____	_____
Which block is yellow?	_____	_____
Which one is the tallest?	_____	_____
Which rock is sharp?	_____	_____
Which dolly has curly hair?	_____	_____
Where, for example, *Where do you sleep?*	_____	_____
Where do you take a bath?	_____	_____
Where do you live?	_____	_____
Where is the red one?	_____	_____
Where is your coat?	_____	_____
Who, for example, *Who drives your car?*	_____	_____
Who do you play with?	_____	_____
Who helps you get dressed?	_____	_____
Who is your best friend?	_____	_____
Who is your teacher?	_____	_____
Whose, for example, *Whose umbrella is that?*	_____	_____
Whose game is that?	_____	_____
Whose baby is Molly?	_____	_____
Whose basketball bounces the best?	_____	_____
Whose house is that?	_____	_____

	Functionally Accurate	Functionally Appropriate
What + do, for example, *What is he doing?*	_____	_____
What is she doing?	_____	_____
What is Daddy doing in the kitchen?	_____	_____
What does Mommy do at work?	_____	_____
What do you like to do outside?	_____	_____
Why, for example, *Why is she crying?*	_____	_____
Why do airplanes fly?	_____	_____
Why do kids go to school?	_____	_____
Why do we have birthday parties?	_____	_____
Why do we use stamps on letters?	_____	_____
When, for example, *When do you eat breakfast?*	_____	_____
When do you take a bath?	_____	_____
When do you go to school?	_____	_____
When do you have a snack?	_____	_____
When does Mommy read to you?	_____	_____
What happened, for example, *What happened to the old shoes?*	_____	_____
What happened to Scott after he fell?	_____	_____
What happened yesterday?	_____	_____
What happened in school today?	_____	_____
What happened on Christmas morning?	_____	_____
Totals	_____	_____

Definitions of response types (from Parnell et al., 1984):

"functionally accurate": "provided factual, acceptable, logical, believable information" (p. 299)

"functionally appropriate": provided "distinctive kind or category of information required by the particular question form" (p. 299).

Using Standardized Tests to Evaluate Language Disorders in Preschoolers

> **WHO?**   SLPs involved in making diagnoses, planning treatment, and evaluating the treatment efficacy of preschool-age children with language disorders.
>
> **WHAT?**   Selecting appropriate standardized tests, tests that provide normative data and prescribe the methods of administration for use with this population.
>
> **WHY?**   To establish eligibility for treatment services or other follow-up measures.
>
> **HOW?**   By carefully reading the manuals that accompany tests on the market, keeping up-to-date with reviews of newer test instruments, and using clinical judgment accrued from your own training and experiences.
>
> **LITERATURE RESOURCES**   See Paul (1995); Weiss, Tomblin, and Robin (1999); and Wyatt (1997).

Given the proliferation of test instruments available to SLPs for purchase, it is advisable for clinicians to have a mental framework to use for the critique of new tests that come on the market. Rarely will we be given the opportunity to spend unlimited funds to purchase new evaluation tools for our clinical test batteries. That being the case, how can we systematically, thoroughly, and accurately make decisions about which tests are likely to be most clinically useful for us? We have to answer this question with an eye toward the demonstrated validity and reliability of the product and not just on the basis of our needing a comprehension measure for preschool-age clients. Following a listing of the characteristics of desirable tests, there will be a summary of general test administration guidelines.

What Are the Characteristics of a Useful Standardized Test to Use with Preschoolers?

❖ Should have engaging, age-appropriate test materials to draw and hold the child's attention.

❖ If pictures are used, they should be clear depictions of the intended exemplars (prototypes).

❖ Manual should offer specific guidance for test scoring and administration.

❖ Some guidance in terms of intervention planning based on the test's results is always appreciated.

❖ Demonstrate sensitivity to cultural differences in terms of test-taking procedures as well as stimuli used. See Wyatt (1997) for an explanation of the biases present in test-taking situations as well as in test materials.

❖ Should be psychometrically sound. This feature was defined and described by McCauley and Swisher (1984).

• McCauley and Swisher (1984) evaluated 30 speech and language tests commonly used with preschoolers and determined that only one met as many as 8 of their 10 criteria for acceptable tests. This situation has improved somewhat over the last 15 years.

- The ten criteria were as follows:
  - an adequate description of the standardization sample
  - a sufficiently large standardization sample
  - item analysis
  - means and standard deviations of performance norms
  - proof of concurrent validity
  - predictive validity
  - test-retest reliability
  - interexaminer reliability
  - adequate description of test administration procedures
  - description of tester qualifications
- Only one test, the then *Test of Language Development* (*TOLD*, 1978), demonstrated as many as eight of the characteristics.
- The remaining tests did not fare well when compared to the ten criteria.
- Over the last several years, a number of popular tests have undergone revision and obvious attention has been paid to shoring up the problems of the second editions. Specifically, changes are evident in:
  - demographics of the standardization sample,
  - performance coefficients have been calculated for subsets of subjects,
  - materials have been examined and altered to eliminate inherent biasing, and
  - test administration directions and rules for interpretation of test results have been altered to eliminate inherent biasing.

A Summary of Considerations for the Selection and Administration of Standardized Tests with Preschool-Age Children

Not just "any available test will do." You have to have a rationale for why you selected a particular test for administration as well as for why you eliminated a test from use.

❖ Many of the tests appropriate for evaluating the preschool-age child have recently been updated. Be sure that you have selected the most recent edition available, for example, *TACL*-3 was published in 1999.

  • Many of these updates were completed to increase the reliability and validity information available for the test as well to expand the tests' utility with nonmajority populations.

❖ Check the demographics of the test's standardization sample and match it to your prospective client before you select it for use. See Vaughn-Cooke (1986) for a summary of the pitfalls of using standardized tests on populations excluded from the normative sample.

❖ Be sure that the test selected matches the child's diagnostic needs. That is, the test should adequately evaluate comprehension competencies if that is what is required. Do not assume that a "Test of Language . . ." necessarily assesses all of the language areas you are interested in.

❖ It is advisable to test both the child's language comprehension and language production abilities, given the relatively better prognosis observed for children who have difficulty with expressive skills only.

❖ Given the limited attention span exhibited by many normally developing preschoolers for test-taking activities, be especially certain that you understand the particular testing conventions for administration and scoring so that you can move through the testing process as quickly as possible.

❖ Learn and use accurate basal and ceiling scoring conventions for each test that you administer.

❖ Test the appropriate age range for the client.

  • If the child's chronological age is close to 5 but it is your observation that his or her abilities are relatively poor when compared with this age expectation, you may select a test that is normally used with children younger than 5 to get a better idea of what the child *can* do rather than what the child *cannot* do.

Clinical Insight

It may be a better idea to consider "developmental age" than chronological age when making decisions about the age-appropriateness of a diagnostic test.

❖ Look carefully for signs early on in testing that the child does not understand the instructions for the test.

  • The child interprets three pictures presented side-by-side as telling one story rather than representing two foils and a correct response.

- Look for perseverative answers, for example, the child always points to the picture at the top-right of the page when shown a set of four pictures.

❖ Be prepared with alternative sets of equivalent test instructions for children with limited comprehension abilities, for example, "We're going to play a copy-cat game and you're gonna do what I do" rather than "I want you to imitate me."

- Another task type that may be used on these tests is the request that the child tell the examiner which pair was the same and which was different. Same/different and judgment tasks ("Which one sounds silly?") should probably not be used until the child is 5 years of age or older because they involve metalinguistic operations that may not be in the repertoire of children prior to that age.

- You will need some general idea of the child's comprehension abilities before you begin.

- Of course, when you make accommodations to directions, you must be sure that they do not compromise the standardization of the test.

- If your directions are very different from the prescribed directions in the test manual, you should explicitly describe these differences in direction-giving in your report.

❖ Give plenty of examples, where permitted, to be sure that the child understands what is expected of him or her. Many standardized tests provide examples. *Use them!*

❖ You can praise children for their performance in terms of the good work they are doing.

- That is, do not praise a child for getting the right answer only.

- Let them know that you appreciate how well they are paying attention.

- Let them know that you appreciate their hard work.

- Unless forbidden as per the test manual, I like to tell preschoolers at the start of testing that some of the work they are going to do will be very easy and some of it will be very hard, and that I just want them to do their best on all of the work.

❖ Watch for signs of fatigue in the child. Many preschool-age children are not used to sitting quietly in adult-directed activities for an hour, let alone longer than that so the noncompliant behaviors you begin to observe as well as the less-than-optimum language performance you record may have more to do with fatigue than typical behavior.

❖ Some negative behaviors that might earn "time outs" in ongoing treatment relationships may have to be ignored in order to ensure that the most information is collected during the limited evaluation time period.

❖ Weigh your choices between gleaning as much information as possible and maintaining the type of behavioral control you would require in ongoing treatment. Admittedly, we sometimes walk a fine line here.

❖ Remember that use of standardized testing means that the language competencies evaluated will be largely *decontextualized*, or taken out of its natural communicative context. For some children this decontextualization is not a familiar experience and their performance on the test may not accurately reflect the extent of their language competence.

❖ Minimize distractions from the task at hand and place extraneous materials beyond the child's reach.

❖ Remember that materials placed on a table surface and manipulated by the child or examiner can make a lot of noise; when using tape recordings or video recordings to check scoring for language information, this noise can be detrimental to accurate transcription.

❖ Sometimes you can earn more cooperation from children if you suggest that they select the next test to be used.

• Be sure, of course, that the order of testing does not matter.

• This choosing often gives children a sense of some control over the proceedings and, when children have a sense of control, they are often more compliant.

Descriptions of Three Tests That Evaluate Both Receptive and Expressive Language Competencies

Here are brief overviews of three commonly used tests that provide diagnostic information for preschool-age children. You will note that the developmental age ranges appropriate for each test represent some overlap.

I. Test of Language Development–Primary–3rd Edition (TOLD-P–3) (1997)

AUTHORS AND PUBLISHER

P. Newcomer and D. Hammill, published by Pro-Ed of Austin, TX.

PURPOSE

❖ This test serves as a linguistically referenced diagnostic tool for children ages 4:0 through 8:11 to:
  • identify children who have difficulty with oral communication
  • identify a child's linguistic strengths and weaknesses
  • document therapeutic progress
  • be useful for research purposes

❖ Nine subtests, six core and three supplementary, covering three linguistic systems (listening, organizing, and speaking) and three linguistic features (semantics, syntax, and phonology) are presented.

❖ Items on each subtest are presented orally or via pictured stimuli.

IMPROVEMENTS OVER PRIOR EDITIONS

❖ There have been many improvements, among them:
  • new stimuli have been drawn
  • new normative data have been collected reflecting results of the 1990 United States Census
  • reliability coefficients reflecting population subgroups have been calculated, among others

SCORES GENERATED

❖ Composite scores (derived from different combinations of subtest results) reflecting the child's abilities for Listening, Organizing, Speaking, Semantics, Syntax, and Spoken Language

❖ In addition, raw scores, age equivalents, percentiles, and standard scores for the individual subtests and quotients for the composites can be determined.

II. Preschool Language Scale-3 (PLS-3) (1992)

AUTHORS AND PUBLISHER

I. Zimmerman, V. Steiner, and R. Pond, published by The Psychological Corporation of San Antonio, TX.

PURPOSE

❖ It serves as a comprehensive test of both receptive and expressive language by presenting subjects with a series of items involving pictured stimuli or manipulated objects.

IMPROVEMENTS OVER PRIOR EDITIONS

❖ According to the manual, this third edition of the test improves upon the first two editions by:

  • providing the examiner with reduced administration time (less than 1 hour)

  • an easier administration process

  • the third edition of the *PLS-3* provides normative data that were collected/ stratified based on the 1980 Census; the standardization sample approached 2000 children and spanned 40 states.

SCORES GENERATED

❖ The *PLS-3* is comprised of two standardized subscales:

  • one for Auditory Comprehension (AC)

  • one for Expressive Communication (EC)

❖ It is appropriate for children ranging in age from birth to 6 years, 11 months.

❖ In addition, this newest version contains three additional measures to be used as supplements where appropriate:

  • an Articulation Screener

  • a Language Sample Checklist

  • a Family Information and Suggestion Form

❖ Administration of the *PLS-3* yields the following scores for both scales:

  • standard score equivalents of the child's raw scores

  • percentile rankings for the standard scores

  • age equivalents for the raw scores

❖ The examiner can also calculate a Total Language standard score and percentile ranking by adding the results of the individual subscales (AC+EC):

  • a Total Language age equivalent can be calculated from the sum of the raw scores from the two subscales (AC+EC).

III. Test of Early Language Development–3rd Edition (TELD-3) (1999)

AUTHORS AND PUBLISHER

W. Hresko, D. Reid, and D. Hammill; published by Pro-Ed, Austin, TX.

PURPOSE

❖ To serve as a measure of receptive and expressive language with particular emphasis on semantics and syntax.

❖ Identification of children who may benefit from early intervention, delineate their language strengths and needs, document progress when early intervention is provided, and provide the clinician with some insights into treatment planning.

❖ Appropriate for children ages 2:0 through 7:11 who speak Standard English and who have been exposed to mainstream American culture. Examiners are cautioned to interpret results with caution if the child does not meet these criteria.

STANDARDIZATION SAMPLE

❖ Over 2200 children representing 35 states served in the standardization sample.

❖ The authors attempted to stratify their sample in terms of national demographics regarding gender, residence, race, geographic region, ethnicity, socioeconomic status, and age according to 1997 U.S. Census data.

TEST AREAS INCLUDED

❖ A diagnostic profile is derived from the child's responses to provide information about performance in both receptive and expressive language as well as in terms of use of semantics and syntax.

TEST ADMINISTRATION

❖ Items are scored as either correct or incorrect, and there are 68 of them, although it is assumed that far fewer than 68 items will be administered given that the test is designed for basal and ceiling scoring.

❖ Pictured stimuli are provided in a separate booklet; all objects needed are included.

SCORES GENERATED

❖ The *TELD-3* yields the following, in addition to the TELD overall Spoken Language score:

  • raw scores
  • percentiles
  • standard scores
  • age equivalents
  • scores for Receptive and Expressive Language subtests

CAUTIONS CONCERNING *TELD-3* LIMITATIONS

❖ Note that the *TELD-3* does not evaluate all aspects of language.

❖ According to the authors, it is important to recognize that some children who have difficulty on this test may just be having difficulty with the particular items on the test and not have a general language problem.

❖ The authors also note that the test is diagnostic in nature in the sense that children with problems can be delineated; however, the test does not, nor was it meant to, give direction for subsequent treatment.

Descriptions of Two Tests That Evaluate Receptive Language Competencies

I. Peabody Picture Vocabulary Test, 3rd Edition (PPVT-III) (1997)

AUTHORS AND PUBLISHER

L. Dunn and L. Dunn, published by American Guidance Service of Circle Pines, MN.

PURPOSE

❖ According to the authors, the *PPVT-III* is designed for persons 2:6 to 90+ years of age.

 • a measure of hearing vocabulary achievement for Standard English

 • the authors note that the test can be used as a screening test of verbal ability

IMPROVEMENTS OVER PRIOR EDITIONS

❖ The third edition includes a number of improvements over earlier editions, including:

 • an increase of test items to 204 for each version of the test (there are two: Form IIIA and Form IIIB)

 • extended national norms both in terms of the ages represented by the sample but also in terms of the geographic and ethnic stratification

 • new stimuli to improve gender and ethnic participation

SCORES GENERATED

❖ Standard scores, percentile rankings, stanines, normal curve equivalents as well as age equivalents can be derived from raw scores.

❖ Confidence bands are also available for the derived scores.

II. Test for Auditory Comprehension of Language, 3rd Edition (TACL-3) (1999)

AUTHOR AND PUBLISHER

E. Carrow-Woolfolk; published by Pro-Ed of Austin, TX.

PURPOSE

❖ To evaluate a child's ability to understand spoken language, specifically in the areas of vocabulary, grammatical morphemes, and elaborated phrases and sentences.

❖ Children are shown pages with colored drawings, three to a page, and asked to point to the picture that best represents what the examiner says.

❖ Normative data are available for children ranging in age from 3:0 through 9:11.

IMPROVEMENTS OVER PRIOR EDITIONS

❖ There is an increase of 22 items on the test, divided among the three subtests.

❖ Following an item analysis of the items in the earlier edition, some items were removed or changed to make them more discriminating.

❖ The normative sample reflects the United States population according to the latest census figures available at the time of publication, with better representation of nonmajority populations.

❖ Reliability coefficients are provided for these subgroups.

SCORES GENERATED

❖ Raw scores, standard scores, percentile ranks, and age equivalents are available.

❖ The sum of the standard scores from all three subtests can, in turn, be converted into a *TACL-3* Quotient.

The Design of a Test Battery for a Child Suspected of a Language Disorder with Rationales for Selection

WHO? SLPs charged with the diagnosis of a young child with a suspected language problem.

WHAT? All clinicians need to be adept at putting together a collection of tests and probes, where needed, to comprehensively evaluate a child's communication problem.

WHY? To appropriately plan a treatment regimen, if one is needed.

HOW? Through collection of preassessment information from a variety of sources and the clinician's own observations and matching the outcome of those observations and the clinician's intuitions with available standardized tests that also match with the child's demographics, for example, race, ethnicity, dominant language, socioeconomic status, and so on.

Here are some questions and issues that should be addressed in the development of an appropriate test battery for a preschool-age child. Notice that the information we have already presented with regard to test selection and the areas of testing that are important for the purposes of differential diagnosis comes into play here.

❖ What is the presenting complaint? Be sure that this issue will be thoroughly covered by the testing you plan to do.

  • Utilize information gleaned from interviews with the primary caregiver(s).

  • Also utilize information gleaned from your own observation as well as the classroom teacher (where relevant), other educators (where relevant), and medical personnel (where relevant).

  • Is there general agreement about the nature of the communication difficulties experienced by the child?

❖ List the features of language that you want to evaluate, for example, semantics and syntax.

  • Do you want to evaluate language comprehension and production?

    – As already noted, evaluation of both receptive and expressive competencies is the wisest course of action.

  • Is there a suspected speech sound disorder?

    – Is the child's speech intelligible?

    – We are less interested in the number of sounds in error than we are in the degree to which the child can make himself or herself understood.

    – Remember to collect both single-word data and a sample of connected speech.

  • Remember that, to evaluate semantics, you must not only assess the child's vocabulary but also the use of a variety of productive semantic relationships.

❖ Select standardized tests that address the questions you want to answer.

- Match up the concerns expressed by others and those delineated from your own observations with available test instruments.

- Will the test's interpretation provide answers to those questions?

- What measures are available, for example, percentile ranking? stanine? age equivalence?

- Remember to check the test's manual for the critical features delineated by McCauley and Swisher (1984). Does the test meet your personal criteria for acceptability with this child?

- Note the language areas assessed. If any are missing, consider the development of a nonstandardized probe to fill in this gap.

- Scan the test for the tasks to be used.

- Will the child understand the instructions as written in the manual? If not make accommodations to them.

- Troubleshoot the tests for bias. Do you have any reason to suspect that the results of the test will be culturally biased for use with this client? If so, can you alter test administration or utilization to eliminate the potential for bias (Vaughn-Cooke, 1986; Wyatt, 1997)?

❖ Consider the practicality of test selection with regard to time allotted for testing.

- If you need to schedule a hearing test and oral mechanism examination in the same session, recognize that these may tax your young client's patience as well.

❖ Consider the practicality of test selection with regard to the child's ability to maintain attention and work at optimum levels during testing.

❖ Study the test manuals in preparation for test administration.

❖ Be sure to arrange the testing in a logical manner.

- If possible, have the hearing testing completed first. This way, if a hearing problem is revealed, you will have the opportunity to compensate for it, or at least consider it, during testing.

- For a child who is reluctant to speak, begin with receptive language tests that require the child to point but not to talk. This may help to boost the child's confidence and develop rapport between client and clinician.

- When reporting the test results, begin by reporting the results of tests and observations that address the presenting complaint to acknowledge the concerns of the individual who referred the child for evaluation.

Clinical Insight

You will undoubtedly notice overlap in the tests you select. This is to be expected, given the make-up of the tests we have available to us for children of preschool age, but it is also desirable to some extent. We should never make a diagnosis based on the results of only one test so the converging data that test overlap provides us is a good thing. Obviously, we do not want our testing to be so redundant that we are basically deriving exactly the same information from a multitude of sources and severely restricting the scope of the information we can glean after our limited evaluation time. When we put together a test battery, we must weigh the benefits of some overlap with our need to manage time in such a way that we can cover relevant language skills and related developmental areas. An example of a test battery for a preschool-age child useful for evaluating language disorders follows.

An Example of a Test Battery Incorporating Standardized and Nonstandardized Tests

❖ Consider the information gleaned from preassessment information to determine what the primary language concern(s) is/are.

❖ Either have the child's hearing tested on site before you begin your evaluation or have recent documentation of the client's hearing acuity levels.

  • Make accommodations in testing procedures as needed.

❖ When possible, observe the child with the primary caregiver(s) in as natural a context as is possible for 5 to 10 minutes.

  • Note interaction patterns for assertiveness and responsiveness of the child in conversation with the primary caregiver(s) versus the clinician, as reported in class by the classroom teacher, and so on.

❖ Select at least one appropriate test in the area of most concern to the referral source, for example, syntax/morphology or vocabulary.

❖ Where possible because of precise preassessment information prepare ahead of time nonstandardized probes that will allow the clinician to fine-tune the evaluation.

  • Other nonstandardized probes will either be developed on line as needed or become a part of diagnostic therapy.

❖ Select a comprehensive language evaluation tool that will provide a comparison between the client's performance and other children in the test's normative sample.

  • Be sure that the test selected is normed on a population that matches the client's age, socioeconomic status, race, and first language.

❖ Be sure that a sufficient language sample has been collected to permit later analysis either during the course of the evaluation or in a separate section of the evaluation.

  • Some of the sample can be used from the interaction between the child and the primary caregiver(s).

  • The language sample corpus can be collected in several clinical settings with several co-conversationalists of differing ages/sizes.

❖ Be sure that the test's purpose fits with the questions you want to answer.

❖ Be sure the test has acceptable reliability and validity measures.

❖ Because few standardized tests permit evaluation of pragmatics, be sure that you have compensated for this through your observation of situations you have contrived for this purpose. Roth and Spekman's (1984a, 1984b) breakdown of pragmatic competencies is utilized.

  • For example, look at the different *communicative functions* the child uses:

    – Engage the child in an activity where insufficient materials are provided. Does the child request assistance? Additional materials? Point out this dilemma to the clinician?

- Look at the child's use of ***presupposition***:
  - Engage the child in a storytelling exercise. Does the child make inappropriate assumptions about your perspective of the story given the information conveyed?
- Look at the child's *conversation skills*:
  - Engage the child in conversation or observe the child in conversation with others. Does the child take turns? Interrupt others? Maintain topics? Initiate topics, and so on?

❖ If concerns were expressed by the referring source or observations were made by the clinician pointing to an anatomical difference affecting language production, perform an oral mechanism exam (see Hall, 1999, for a comprehensive description of this technique adapted for young children and adults).

Use of Dynamic Assessment Techniques with Preschool-Age Children

WHO? SLPs should attempt to include some dynamic assessment strategies when performing language evaluations with preschool-age children.

WHAT? Dynamic assessment techniques determine the type of support, for example, stimulus, feedback, or reinforcement, the child needs in order to successfully complete a language task or demonstrate a language competency.

WHY? Information gleaned through dynamic assessment can help to bridge the gap between assessment and intervention by determining the specific therapeutic techniques that are likely to be successful.

HOW? Utilize the diagnostic session as well as several sessions of diagnostic therapy, if a disorder is revealed, to manipulate teaching strategies so that the most effective techniques for the child can be determined.

LITERATURE RESOURCES Bain and Olswang (1995); Lidz and Peña (1996); Olswang and Bain (1991); Olswang, Bain, and Johnson (1992).

The suggestions that follow should help the clinician gain some insights into how a young child with a language disorder may best learn language. What cues appear to be the most salient to the child and how can treatment be configured to maximize the use of those cues?

Clinical Insight

Dynamic assessment is to some extent old wine in a new bottle. It seems to me that it is a hybrid between what we have traditionally called "diagnostic therapy" and nonstandardized assessment. Its purpose reflects a Vygotskian perspective, that is, how do we answer the question: "What kind of support must I give this child so that she or he can be successful with this task?" Besides the focus on the child's success, focus is placed on how the child is learning and what we can do to facilitate that learning, rather than on the specific language element the child can produce. Said another way, the focus is on teaching and not testing. This is closely associated with Vygotsky's notion of the Zone of Proximal Development (ZPD) or "ZOPED"; the ZPD is the area between the point where the child can function competently with support and the point where the child functions without the support provided by the clinician.

❖ Recognize that therapy is comprised of several manipulable components including how we provide stimuli, feedback, and reinforcement or motivation to our clients.

❖ When we determine the type of stimuli we will use, we are considering changes we can apply to:

 • the directions or tasks we give, for example, do we ask a question or do we provide a "fill-in"? Do we tell the child to pay attention?

- the type of materials we use, for example, three-dimensional objects versus two-dimensional pictures, supportive objects for prompts when we ask the child to explain a process; and

- the frequency and type of prompts and cues we use, for example, do we provide an oral model for the correct answer or do we provide a written prompt? Maybe we will provide a number of prompts including auditory, visual, and even tactile cues.

❖ Although most of the literature focuses on changes in stimuli when referring to dynamic assessment, I believe that feedback, the information we provide our clients about the adequacy of their performance, also has an effect on the child's ability to learn.

- Explicit feedback versus implicit feedback?

- Initial provision of feedback or feedback only after the child has made an attempt to judge his or her own performance.

- Manipulations of feedback provision should enhance a child's development of self-monitoring behaviors.

❖ Again, although it is not the classic view of dynamic assessment, I believe that reinforcement, or the type of motivation we provide our young clients to consistently try their best and repeat an acceptable performance, is also part of dynamic assessment.

- We want to know what type of reinforcement is necessary to motivate the child to perform at an optimum level.

  - Is any tangible reinforcement needed?

  - Does praise work successfully as a reinforcer?

  - When the task is a functional one, is the child's success at communicating serving as an effective reinforcer?

❖ Experiment during the course of the evaluation with manipulating the extent and type of stimulus support, feedback, and reinforcement provided and note carefully how the child performs. That is, what is helpful? What is necessary? What may hinder independent performance?

❖ Dynamic assessment is a particularly useful approach when working with the culturally and linguistically different child because, as we focus on how learning is aided rather than on what the child knows, we remove much of the language biasing from our tasks.

General Principles for Collecting a Language Sample From a Preschool-Age Child

WHO? Speech-language pathologists should be prepared to collect a *representative* language sample from all young children and analyze it.

WHAT? Strategies and techniques for the collection, analysis, and interpretation of language samples.

WHY? Language sample analysis is important to make inferences about a child's underlying knowledge of the language system. That is, by looking at language performance (the corpus of utterances collected), we can infer the child's language competence.

HOW? Various techniques are available for collecting a valid (representative) sample. Most techniques attempt to facilitate the child's production of contextualized utterances, that represent the typical language output of the child. Thus, situations that are truly communicative are often employed.

LITERATURE RESOURCES See specific techniques and procedures delineated by the following:

Hughes, D., McGillivray, L., & Schmidek, M. (1997). *Guide to narrative language: Procedures for assessment.* Eau Claire: WI: Thinking Publications.

Lund, N., & Duchan, J. (1993). *Assessing children's language in naturalistic contexts* (3rd ed.). Englewood Cliffs, NJ: Prentice Hall.

Miller, J. (1981). *Assessing language production in children: Experimental procedures.* Needham Heights, MA: Allyn & Bacon.

Paul, R. (1995). *Language disorders from infancy through adolescence: Assessment and intervention.* St. Louis: Mosby-Year Book, Inc.

Retherford-Stickler, K. (1993). *Guide to analysis of language transcripts* (2nd ed.). Eau Claire, WI: Thinking Publications.

Given the importance of the language sample in the diagnostic process, I think it is important to be sure to justify all of the different measures that can be derived from a well-collected, representative sample. Here are some ideas.

❖ Language samples potentially provide clinicians and others with a rich database from which many language features can be evaluated.

❖ Although language sample collection is often viewed as a prodigious undertaking, the information it yields generally makes up for the outlay of time on the front end of the process.

❖ Language samples are versatile sources of information and can be used to closely look at the following.

• Child's use of pragmatics, including:

– speech acts

– communicative intents

– presupposition

– conversation parameters, for example, assertiveness, responsiveness

- Child's use of semantics, including:
  - semantic relations
  - vocabulary size
  - lexical diversity
- Child's use of morphology, including:
  - use of grammatical morphemes
  - use of derivational morphemes
- Child's use of syntax, including:
  - use of different sentence structures, for example, declaratives, interrogatives, imperatives
  - use of clause structures, for example, embedding and conjoining
- Child's use of phonology, including:
  - How intelligible is the child?
  - Does intelligibility differ between single-word productions and connected speech?
  - use of phonological rules and phonotactic constraints
  - use of phonological patterns or processes
- Child's use of extralinguistic communication features, including:
  - use of gesture, for example, eye gaze, hands, head movements
  - use of suprasegmental features, for example, stress, prosodic contours
  - use of metalinguistic knowledge to determine the adequacy of the messages sent and received

❖ How long should a sample be?

- Language samples need to be large enough to represent the entire corpus of utterances the child is capable of producing, but small enough to be collected and analyzed in a reasonable amount of time.

- For diagnostic purposes, we generally collect 50 to 100 utterances. The size of the sample is almost secondary to the faith of the clinician in its *representativeness*. So, a smaller representative sample is better than a larger but questionable sample.
  - Miller (1981) suggests that samples should be carefully scanned for inclusion of rote-learned passages, many imitated utterances, songs or nursery rhymes, and other minimally processed speech and language.
  - When samples contain substantive proportions (more than 25%) of rote-learned or minimally processed/generated language, these sections should be eliminated and additional, more spontaneous utterances added to the corpus where possible.

- Note that different analysis techniques call for different sample, or *corpus*, sizes. For example:
  - Lee (1974), the author of the Developmental Sentence Scoring technique (DSS), recommended samples of 50 utterances; normative data provided for the DSS are based on the collection of samples of that length.

- Brown (1973) based his normative data for Mean Length of Utterance (MLU) on samples of 100 utterances.

- Miller and Chapman's (1981) additional MLU normative data were based on samples of 50 utterances.

❖ How are language samples collected? There are several considerations including materials used, who should serve as a conversation partner, topics of conversation, recording materials, where the sample is collected, and so forth.

Clinical Insight

The goal is to collect a sample, or subset, of all the utterances a child can produce and then make inferences from that to what the child's entire repertoire must be. If we want to use Chomsky's distinction between language performance and language competence, we can view our sampling process as using language performance to make inferences about a child's underlying language competence.

❖ The suggestions that follow describe a sample collected in the best of all possible worlds, meaning that it may not always be feasible to take all of these factors into consideration due to time available for data collection and logistical constraints.

- Materials

  - Select materials that are developmentally appropriate in terms of both the cognitive skills needed and the motor skills needed.

  - If the child has any physical limitations, take these into account when selecting materials.

  - Create situations with materials where meaningful information needs to be conveyed. For example, what is likely to happen if you ask a child to complete a project but do not provide the child with sufficient materials?

  - Use a combination of *familiar* and *unfamiliar* toys or games. Familiar toys brought into an evaluation setting with a new clinician create an information "mismatch" where it makes sense for the child to share information. Unfamiliar toys and games make it more likely that the child will ask the clinician for information.

  - Consider use of "provocative" toys. Miller (1981) suggests that using broken toys, for example, trucks without wheels or dolls missing a limb to facilitate question asking, especially Why? and How? questions by the child.

- Conversation partners

  - The most representative language samples will be collected when children have the opportunity to interact with a number of different conversation partners.

  - To better ensure a representative sample, collect data (spontaneous utterances) during the child's interaction with familiar adults (family members and/or child care workers) who know the child's linguistic capabilities as well as with adults unfamiliar with the child's language (the clinician) and other children.

  – The selection of children as conversation partners ideally should include same-age peers, more than one other child (so that triadic as well as dyadic interactions are collected), and children who are both familiar and unfamiliar to the child.

  – Normally developing children often demonstrate different conversation styles with different conversation partners.

  – These differences manifest themselves as differences in who contributes more to the conversation in terms of new topics (topic initiation), number of turns, and length of turns as well as in the sophistication of those turns.

  – Some conversation partners are more dominant in conversations, or **assertive** (Fey, 1986), leaving their partners less room to be assertive but possibly with more opportunities to be **responsive** to their partners' requests.

  – Differences in linguistic sophistication will also yield differences in conversation contributions. Accommodations to the less-sophisticated partner may include simplified vocabulary and syntax as well as dominance in controlling the topic selection of the conversation. It is important to know if the child perceives the need to make these accommodations and can make them.

• Topics of conversation

  – Do some planning ahead of time to anticipate conversation topics that are not only developmentally appropriate, but also fit the interests of the child.

  – Topics of conversation may be suggested by the clinician, the child's primary caregiver(s), classroom teachers, or the child.

  – They may be supported by the use of materials (see the preceding Materials section) or there may not be supportive materials used in conjunction with their discussion. For younger children, supportive materials may be essential to collection of a sample. For example, if "making popcorn" is the topic of interest, having popcorn-making paraphernalia available to provide context support may facilitate discussion.

• Collection of the sample

  – Videotaping of samples is preferable to audiotaping alone. Unfortunately, the videotaping of a sample is not always feasible.

  – Be sure to include sufficient context notes during the time of sample collection. That is, be sure to document the situations in which language production took place. Ideally, you will be recording not just what the child produced, but also the linguistic and nonlinguistic contexts that preceded and followed that production.

  – For each child utterance, answer the questions:

  What was said before the child's utterance?

What was said after the child's utterance?

What materials did the child have during the utterance?

What gestures, if any, accompanied the utterance?

Was the utterance spontaneous?

Was the utterance elicited? If so, how?

Was the utterance a partial or complete imitation?

What was the child's communicative intent(s)?

– Be aware that, if you are videotaping the sample, the introduction of a camera, whether or not the camera is operated from inside the data collection room, can be obtrusive and result in the collection of a sample that is not representative of typical interactions between the participants.

– Ask the parent or caregiver if the sample collected was typical of the language that the child produces in a more natural setting.

– Use a high-quality tape recorder if videotaping equipment is not available.

– Many clinics have FM microphones that can be worn by the child or the clinician to increase the fidelity of the signal produced. Of course, this should make transcription more accurate.

– FM microphones should be used with care. Their placement, especially if clipped to a child's clothing, may cause muffled recordings if the child fidgets and the microphone becomes obstructed. In some instances, having the clinician wear the microphone allows for a more predictable signal.

• Elicitation techniques

– Ideally, we want the utterances produced to be spontaneous in nature. That is, we want the productions to be part of play, being sensitive to the child's willingness to interact with us. You may need to attempt this maneuver several times before conversational interaction begins.

– Remember that if the child prefers to talk about what he or she is doing and not interact with the examiner, per se, those utterances can also be used.

– Do not bombard the child with questions. To elicit more language, use open-ended comments when possible. For example, say "I wonder how the truck got all the way down there" or "How did the truck get there?" rather than "Where's the truck?"

– Questions are useful because they *signal that the child can take a turn* and, because *they actually turn the floor over to the child* so they should be used but not overused!

– One key for "overuse" of questions is: Does the child appear to be in the process of interrogation?

– Note that some of the question types used will inherently limit the language output of the answer, for example, "What's this? Is this a ducky?"

– Choice questions are sometimes useful with reticent children because they provide the child with an opportunity to be right, for example, "Is this a grape or an orange?" "Do you like ice cream or apple pie best?" "Do you think the boy is happy or sad?"

• Where is the sample collected?

  – Collecting samples in the child's home can have the added benefit of being a familiar and presumably safer place than an unfamiliar clinic or school room. So, the child may be more willing to interact. Also, the clinician will be able to observe what the language demands are for the child in the home environment.

  – Collecting samples at home can also be more distracting for the child due to the presence of other family members and siblings, and offer less control for the clinician in terms of noise, lighting, materials, and behavior management.

  – Consider having the primary caregiver(s) collect some of the language sample at home with the clinician not present during activities of daily living.

  – Family members need to be trained to write down what the child says, what they believe the child meant, as well as the context for the utterance. Special forms can be provided to facilitate language sample collection.

  – Collecting samples in the child's preschool classroom or day care center may have logistic complications because usually the clinician will need to be in the classroom itself and distractions may result from unwanted participation by other children.

  – Collecting samples in a classroom environment will also provide the clinician with some insight into the language demands placed on the child in the classroom and will provide a more natural environment for collecting information about how the child interacts with classmates.

  – Consider having classroom teachers and/or aides collect some of the language sample data from the classroom environment.

  – The clinician will need to train these individuals to write down what the child says, what they believe the child meant, and what the context was for the utterance. Special forms can be provided to the classroom personnel to facilitate language sample collection.

  – Remember that data collected in a clinic environment or in a school therapy room is not being collected in a highly natural context. We cannot discount the effect that unfamiliarity may play in the quality and quantity of language collected.

❖ Some special circumstances require accommodations to the language sampling procedure.

  • Highly unintelligible children

    – Use a more supportive set of stimulus materials that will yield a *closed set* of utterances rather than using techniques, usually conversation, that will result in an *open set* of utterances. A closed set provides you with more predictability.

    – Repeat what the child has said, or rather, what you *think* the child has said. This approach serves several purposes. First, it tends to jog the examiner's mind about the context as well as content of the sample. Second, it serves to aid the transcriber in terms of accuracy of post hoc transcription. And third, this often gives the child the opportunity to correct the examiner and clarify errors of transcription, for example, "No, I said 'He wasn't sleepy.'"

– Whether video- or audiotaping, be sure to use a lot of reiteration of the child's productions as well as your own interpretations of what you believe the child means. This will be invaluable when you attempt to transcribe the tape.

– Use a story retelling task, where the child is first read a story where target words and sounds are embedded, and then the child is asked to tell the story back to the clinician or another listener. Again, the use of supportive materials is useful to ensure a closed set of productions, decreasing the likelihood that immature memory skills are responsible for the child's performance.

– Do not assume that children will understand the word *story*, as in "Tell me a story." Instead, use the phrase, "Once upon a time . . ." and with your intonation indicate that the child is supposed to complete the sentence.

• Very reticent children

– All of the suggestions given above for the child with a hearing impairment are valid here as well.

– Often, children with language impairments are reticent and they offer very little spontaneous language. Their samples take considerably longer to collect. In this case, a number of techniques can be tried.

– When you are attempting to establish rapport with the child for sample collection purposes, be sure to accept the child's gestural communication as valid turn taking, at least at first. Remember that in many adult-to-adult conversations, gestures are often perfectly appropriate, given the conversation context. Of course, if the child is capable of producing verbal language, you will want to record this.

Miller's (1981) Suggestions for Clinicians Gathering a Language Sample

These suggestions, reprinted in the 1992 edition of *Language Sample Analysis: The Wisconsin Guide* (Leadholm & Miller, pp. 17–18), focus on how a clinician can establish and maintain an interaction with a child that will yield useful information about the child's communicative competencies.

❖ Be enthusiastic.

❖ Be patient.

❖ Listen and follow the child's lead.

❖ Value the child.

❖ Do not play the fool.

❖ Learn to think like a child.

Miller (1981) also suggested that there are at least four different approaches or styles one can use with young children to assist in getting the young, reticent child ready for the language sampling session. The approach that is most appropriate will vary depending on the child's cognitive level and temperament.

❖ For the child who is self-conscious about his or her communication difficulties with talking, *say nothing* for at least 5 minutes after greeting the child so that the child feels no immediate pressure to converse.

❖ Use *parallel play* with little accompanying talking during the first few minutes of your interaction. Miller suggests that the child with cognitive functioning at 30 months or less will match up best with this approach.

❖ With the child whose cognitive level is between 3 and 5 years of age, *interactive play* with little accompanying talking for several minutes is usually most appropriate.

❖ For children between 3 and 9 years of age, interactive play can often be utilized successfully where the clinician and the child work cooperatively with some activity.

• At the beginning of an interaction, talking should be directed at toys, not the child.

Analysis of Language Samples: General and Specific Guidelines

Once you have collected your representative language sample, it will be important to analyze the language data in the most efficient and effective manner. Obviously, you have to have some idea about the sorts of information that will be most useful to you. That is, if you are primarily concerned, for example, with the child's use of pragmatic aspects of language, your language sample should include analysis of communicative intents, use of presupposition, and discourse rules (Roth & Spekman, 1984a). Here are some practical, and general, suggestions to follow in the analysis of your sample. Following these general guidelines, there will be specific suggestions for how to analyze your sample when your interests focus on one or another area of language.

General Guidelines

❖ Transcribe your sample as soon after collecting it as possible utilizing the context notes you included when collecting the sample data. It will surprise you how much you can remember shortly after sample collection that fades from memory several days later.

❖ Broad transcription is generally sufficient unless there is a particular reason why narrow transcription would be more useful for the clinician's decision making.

❖ Evaluate the representativeness of the sample and consider elimination of lengthy passages of rote-learned material, directly imitated utterances, and utterances otherwise constrained by adult input, for example, Yes-No questions addressed by an adult to the child.

❖ Reevaluate the size of the sample after eliminating those portions deemed unrepresentative. Will it be necessary to collect additional language sample data? Are you using a particular analysis that requires a certain number of utterances in order to use their normative data? If so, additional sample collection definitely will be required.

❖ Select an analysis type from all possibilities that is appropriate for the client. Do not underestimate or overestimate the child's ability by choosing the wrong analysis type and risk losing important data.

  • Is the analysis type appropriate for the child's developmental language level? For example, if the child is producing examples of complex sentences, you probably would not want to focus on an analysis of semantic relationships because of the risk of underestimating the child's ability.

  • Conversely, if the child is primarily producing single-word utterances, an analysis that focuses on simple sentence production would fail to capture the lexical diversity that might be present in the child's sample.

❖ Again, pay careful attention to the context notes that you prodigiously wrote during the sample's collection so that you can be more certain that, for example, your analysis of word meanings matches the child's intended meaning and not the typical adult's. That is, a word such as "up" may signify an action word/verb for a child although it appears to be a locative/preposition for an adult.

Specific Examples of Language Sample Analyses

❖ Analysis of semantic/lexical development

- Delineate examples of substantive versus relational words (Bloom, 1973).

- Delineate the presence of different semantic relationships, for example, Agent + Object, as per Brown (1973). See Retherford, Schwartz, and Chapman (1981) for a delineation of semantic roles and relationships in mother-child interactions.

- Calculate a type/token ratio: What is the proportion of the number of *different* words produced in a sample divided by the total number of words used by the child in the sample? See Miller (1981); Retherford (1993); and Templin (1957) for a database for comparison and information about interpretation of this measure of lexical diversity.

- For "first vocabularies," utilize a taxonomy like Nelson's (1973) or Benedict's (1979) and delineate the word categories used by the child. Be able to answer the following:

  - Is the child using both specific and general nominals?

  - Is the child using words to signify actions?

  - Is the child using personal-social words?

  - Is the child using words to modify?

  - Are pronouns used?

  - Are formulas used, for example, "gimmedat"?

- Question the child's use of both receptive and expressive vocabulary.

- Use checklists such as those provided by the *MacArthur Communication Development Inventories* (Fenson et al., 1993) to supplement information gleaned from language sample collection. These have been shown to be valid when used with children older than 30 months whose vocabularies are delayed (Thal, Bates, Goodman, & John-Cembalo, 1997).

❖ Syntax/Morphology: Brown's 14 Grammatical Morphemes, Mean Length of Utterance (MLU), and Developmental Sentence Scoring (DSS)

- Use a checklist of Brown's 14 Grammatical Morphemes to determine which of these morphemes has been acquired by the child (90% usage in obligatory contexts).

- Determine which of the 14 grammatical morphemes are emerging in the child's expressive repertoire (present less than 90% of the time).

- These grammatical morphemes normally *begin to emerge* at around 18 months of age when children are beginning to enter Brown's Stage II.

- See Miller (1981) for a useful suggestion for delineating the presence and appropriateness of the 14 grammatical morphemes within a sample.

- The 14 morphemes of interest are:

  - present progressive (-*ing*)

  - prepositions *in* and *on*

  - regular plural (-*s*)

- irregular past (e.g., *drove*) and regular past (*-ed*)
- possessive (*-'s*)
- articles (*a, the*)
- uncontractible and contractible copulas (e.g., *am, is, are*)
- uncontractible and contractible auxiliaries (e.g., *am, is, are*)
- regular and irregular third-person verbs (*-s*)

Clinical Insight

When using the terms "uncontractible" and "contractible," Brown did not mean "uncontracted" and "contracted." He was referring to whether or not the copula or auxiliary form could be contracted or was not contractible in that structure, not whether it was or was not. Thus, in the sentence "He is ready," the copula form *is* represents an uncontracted, but *contractible* copula form.

- Mean Length of Utterance is probably the most commonly used measure of utterance length and complexity when used as a measure of the average number of morphemes per utterance. Its validity as a measure of complexity diminishes beyond an MLU of 4.00.

  - Original data for MLU were published by Brown (1973) based on only three children, and gleaned from 100-utterance samples.

  - Subsequent data were published by Miller and Chapman (1981) for 123 children ranging in age from 17 to 59 months; these data were based on 50-utterance samples.

  - Leadholm and Miller (1992) published MLU data for 266 children ranging in age from 3 to 13 years of age.

  - Lists of rules for counting morphemes and calculating MLU can be found in a number of resources (Owens, 1996; Retherford, 1993) all adapted or reprinted from the original delineation in Brown (1973).

- Developmental Sentence Scoring (DSS) (Lee, 1974) provides a systematic developmental analysis of eight grammatical categories, for example, noun modifiers, personal pronouns, main verbs, secondary verbs, negatives, conjunctions, interrogative reversals, and Wh-questions, based on a sample of 50 sentences (utterances must contain a subject and a predicate).

  - Remember that not all language features nor even all syntactic structures/morphological markers are evaluated using this procedure.

  - Utterances not meeting this criterion (subject + predicate) are viewed as presentence utterances and do not qualify for DSS analysis; instead they qualify for Developmental Sentence Types analysis for presentence utterances, which is now rarely used.

  - Sentences earn points according to the developmental level of the exemplars of the grammatical category used as well as an extra point (the "sentence point"), if the sentence meets all adult grammatical, semantic, and pragmatic constraints.

– Lee's text provides numerical equivalents for productions and descriptions of potential examples.

– Normative data are provided from a small sample of middle-class children ages 2:3 to 6:6 from the Evanston, Illinois, area delineated at the 10th, 25th, 50th, 75th, and 90th percentile. SLPs are able to extrapolate their particular client's percentile performance and calculate approximate age equivalences.

– Children falling more than one full point below the 10th percentile for their age are the most likely candidates for intervention.

– Clinicians can look for the following in addition to the total DSS and projected age equivalence and can use them as criterion-referenced measures when subsequently retesting the child:

→ Did the child produce examples in all categories or are some columns representing the grammatical categories blank?

→ What are the individual developmental levels for each of the eight grammatical categories?

→ What was the developmental score for any forms or structures unsuccessfully attempted by the child?

→ How many of the utterances produced by the child during sample collection qualified for DSS analysis (subject + predicate)?

→ How many sentences earned the extra sentence point?

– See Weiss (1983) for some additional examples of sentence scoring using Lee's Developmental Sentence Scoring conventions that may help the novice with this analysis.

❖ Pragmatic Analysis: Look at the child's understanding of the parameters of conversation; utilize assertiveness/responsiveness analysis

• The sample you have collected can also be analyzed in terms of the communicative intentions you have observed the child use either spontaneously or within more contrived situations.

– Use Coggins and Carpenter's (1981) set of eight communicative intentions as a first taxonomy for analyzing the intentions of very young and/or very reticent children.

– Delineate whether the child is using verbal, or nonverbal means, or a combination of the two when conveying these intentions.

– Is the child's range of communicative intentions limited? Extensive?

– In cases where words are being used to enact a communicative intent, is the child relegated to one word per intention or does the child use a variety of words?

• The sample can also be used to investigate the child's use of conversation bids that can be considered assertive or responsive as per Fey (1986).

– To be assertive and responsive is to understand the basic rules of conversation use: you initiate interactions with statements or questions without being asked to do so (assertiveness) and you respond when requested to do so (responsiveness).

– Samples can be analyzed on the sentence level by first coding the utterances (see Fey, 1986, for a description of the coding categories). Once coded, you can calculate at least two basic measures:

→ Number of assertives produced by the child divided by the total number of assertives produced in the conversation is equal to the relative assertiveness of the child in that conversation.

→ Number of responses made by the child divided by the number of requests for response made by the conversation partner.

– Note that the utilization of different co-conversationalists may yield different ratios; that is, different co-conversationalists take more or less control of conversations. Ratios close to .50 indicate that the conversation is being handled in an egalitarian manner.

– A discourse-level analysis can also be done using Fey's taxonomy to analyze the child's ability and/or willingness to initiate and maintain topics.

– See the following more detailed description of Fey's (1986) model.

• The sample can also be used to check for examples of the child's ability to take the perspective of the listener by demonstrating accurate presuppositional abilities.

– Does the child ever make changes in how he speaks or what he says to accommodate the needs of the listener?

– Does the child appear to be aware that not everyone shares the same background knowledge of a topic, possesses differences in linguistic competencies, or possesses different status as speakers and accommodate for those differences?

– Is the child able to respond differently when requested to clarify what was said?

– How extensive a repertoire did the child demonstrate of successful strategies for clarification?

→ Does the child recognize the need for clarification without prompting?

→ Does the child use lexical replacement, or addition of words, or deletion of words to provide the listener with clarification?

❖ Phonological development can also be assessed via a spontaneous language sample.

• Some investigators believe it is the most valid way to collect speech sound data because the information is in a connected or coarticulated format.

• Given the careful measures taken to collect and analyze a valid language sample, it makes sense to get as much diagnostic use from it as possible.

• Additional resource guides will describe precise methodologies for analysis of a child's speech sounds, but, for our purposes, the most important judgment to make is whether the child's speech is intelligible enough to be understood by conversation partners unfamiliar with the child.

• Is there a significant difference between the child's intelligibility when saying single words and when producing connected speech?

- Can you best describe the child's intelligibility by answering one of the following questions affirmatively?

  – Is the child intelligible most of the time?

  – Is the child intelligible most of the time although speech errors are noticeable?

  – Is the child intelligible if the topic is known?

  – Is the child often unintelligible even if the context of the conversation is known?

  – Is the child often so difficult to understand that ongoing communication is difficult?

  – Is the child rarely intelligible, even in single words?

- If intelligibility is compromised, it will be necessary to do a more thorough analysis.

  – An independent analysis, where the child's sound productions are not related to an adult standard (e.g., "What sounds can this child produce?")

  – A relational analysis, where the child's sound productions are related to the adult standard (e.g., "How correct are the sounds produced by the child?")

- Using developmental information about phoneme acquisition (see Smit et al., 1990), determine whether the child is not producing sounds that are typically produced by children at that age.

- If the child demonstrates multiple sound errors, are they related by place and/or manner of articulation?

- Can the sound errors be described as the result of phonological processes or simplification patterns that are commonly observed in young, preschool-age children (see Stoel-Gammon & Dunn, 1985; Preisser, Hodson, & Paden, 1988).

Computerized Analysis of Language Transcripts

WHO?   SLPs and others who want to be able to quickly analyze language sampling transcripts.

WHAT?   Analyses via computer program allow the clinician to streamline the format of the analyses to provide the most useful information relevant to clinical questions.

WHY?   Software technology allows clinicians to provide data to caregivers and other referral sources soon after the data are collected. This may cut down on the lag time between the evaluation session and the development of goals, as well as the implementation of a treatment program.

WHEN?   The analyses can be run following input of the data.

HOW?   See descriptions of three analysis systems designed by MacWhinney and Snow (1995) (CHILDES); Miller and Chapman (1993) (SALT); and Long, Fey, and Channell (2000) (Computerized Profiling); see the following.

I think that it is very important that the use of a computerized system does not serve as an excuse for avoiding careful study and understanding of the analyses they perform. That is, your ability to interpret the data analyses is dependent upon your ability to understand the procedures inherent in the analyses.

Clinical Insight

Some of the now-computerized programs represent analyses that clinicians have been performing by hand for years, for example, DSS. As any veteran user of DSS can tell you, there are many different ways to use the data gleaned from the analysis protocol in addition to the calculation of the DSS itself, such as which categories have no representation, the average developmental levels calculated for each of the eight categories, and the proportion of sentences earning sentence points from sample to sample. Thus, the DSS score itself does not tell the whole story. The novice who is only familiar with the computer technique may miss this information.

❖ The Child Language Data Exchange System (CHILDES) represents a sizable database of language samples of children's conversations with and without their caregivers.

   • The purpose of the exchange is to allow researchers to easily download samples collected by other investigators for use as a corpus for answering their own language queries.

   • Analysis tools include the Codes for the Human Analysis of Transcripts (CHAT) that provide conventions for the transcription and coding of samples.

   • Computerized Language Analysis or CLAN represents a package of programs to analyze the samples coded according to CHAT conventions.

- Additional information can be obtained from the following resources:
  - MacWhinney, B. (1995). *The CHILDES-Project: Tools for Analyzing Talk* (2nd ed.). Hillsdale: NJ: Lawrence Erlbaum.
  - http://www.psy.cmu.edu/childes
  - Brian MacWhinney, Ph.D., Department of Psychology, Carnegie-Mellon University, Pittsburgh, PA 15213
  - Enroll in an electronic (e-mail) mailing list posting information regarding updates, additions to the database, and so on, by sending mail to info-childes-request@andrew.cmu.edu.

❖ Systematic Analysis of Language Transcripts (SALT)

- Developed by Professors Jon Miller and Robin Chapman at the Language Analysis Laboratory at the University of Wisconsin–Madison.
- Contact them for further information:
  - salt@waisman.wisc.edu
  - http://www.waisman.wisc.edu/salt/
  - Phone: (608) 263-6791; FAX: (608) 263-7710
  - Waisman Research Center, University of Wisconsin–Madison, 1500 Highland Avenue, Madison, WI 53705-2280.
- According to the Web site, SALT "contains the basic tools needed to transcribe language samples into a common format, to compute a series of general analyses of lexical, syntactic, semantic, pragmatic, rate, fluency, and error categories, and to compare individual transcripts to a reference database of age-matched peers."
- A nonexhaustive list of more specific sample analyses provided:
  - type-token ratio
  - frequency, length, rate of pauses
  - distribution of speaker turns by length
  - MLU and Brown's linguistic stage
  - frequencies for any specified set of words, such as question words
- Results can be compared with a corpus of normative data collected from 250+ children ranging in age from 3 to 13 years.
- Formats compatible with PCs and Apple Macintosh computers are available.

❖ Computerized Profiling (CP)

- Originally developed by Steven Long, now affiliated with Case Western Reserve University, and Marc Fey, now at the University of Kansas Medical Center, in the middle 1980s.
- CP is now freeware; therefore, it can be downloaded and used without restriction from the authors.
- It represents a series of programs that can analyze either orthographically or phonetically transcribed samples.

- An overview of the programs and information on downloading them for personal use can be found at http://www.cwru.edu/artsci/cosi/faculty/long/research/info/info.htm

- Its programs can help the clinician analyze information in the areas of semantics, grammar, narrative development, pragmatics (specifically conversation acts), and phonology/prosody.

- Many of the specific programs available through CP are based on other published analysis procedures, for example:

  - *Language Assessment, Remediation, and Screening Procedure* (*LARSP*), Crystal, Fletcher, and Garman (1989).

  - *Index of Productive Syntax* (*IPSyn*), Scarborough (1990).

  - *Profile of Phonology* (*PROPH*), based on Crystal (1982); Grunwell (1987); and others.

Assessment of Children's Use of Their Language Competencies

> **WHO?**   SLPs evaluating preschool-age children with language disorders.
>
> **WHAT?**   Children with language disorders present with a great deal of variety in terms of how they actually use the language that they have.
>
> **WHY?**   SLPs want to select the most efficacious treatment approach for their preschool-age clients and the child's pattern of language use provides insight into this selection.
>
> **HOW?**   Determine children's relative use of assertive conversation acts and the degree to which they are responsive to their conversation partners.
>
> **LITERATURE RESOURCE** See Fey (1986).

What follows is an interesting pragmatics-based perspective that represents one way of conceptualizing a bridge between assessment and intervention for young children with language disorders. You will notice right away that the focus is not on the quantification of a child's language competencies, for example, syntax measures, but on the quality of how the child actually uses the language repertoire that he or she has acquired in conversation contexts.

❖ Children may differ in their recognition that they need to be both assertive and responsive in conversations (Fey, 1986).

  • Assertiveness refers to the ability and/or willingness to provide unsolicited conversational bids, such as comments and requests for information.

  • Responsiveness refers to the ability and/or willingness to provide appropriate responses to request forms directed to the child, for instance, responses to requests for information and responses to requests for clarification.

❖ Using these two parameters, Fey (1986) delineated four patterns of language use:

  • "Active conversationalists" are both assertive and responsive.

  • "Passive conversationalists" are responsive but not assertive.

  • "Inactive communicators" are not assertive or responsive.

  • "Verbal noncommunicators" are assertive but not responsive.

❖ Analysis of children's conversational samples with a variety of co-conversationalists will yield information regarding the child's ability to demonstrate assertiveness and responsiveness.

Clinical Insight

It is important to remember that children will behave differently in conversations depending on who their conversation partner or partners are. Differences in status may lead to very different profiles of assertive and responsive behaviors. Children interacting with their preschool-age peers may demonstrate the ability to hold their own in a conversation, but may show far less in the way of assertive conversation behaviors when in conversation with a teacher or parent. That is why a variety of samples must be collected before determining a child's status as far as use "type" is concerned.

❖ Fey (1986, pp. 72–73) delineated a taxonomy of assertive and responsive conversational acts to describe performance at the sentence level.

  • Utterances can be coded as assertive, responsive, imitations, or "other."

  • The assertive and responsive categories are further divided into types.

    – Assertives: requests, comments, disagreements, and performatives

    – Requestives: responses to requests for action or attention

❖ Discourse-level performance can also be analyzed using this taxonomy, for example, topic manipulation.

❖ Determination of the child's pattern can be calculated by looking at ratios of assertive and responsive utterances produced by the participants.

❖ Not every child fits neatly into one of the four patterns.

❖ An example of each follows.

  • Measure of assertiveness

    – Total number of assertive utterances produced by a child, divided by the total number of assertive utterances produced in the conversation, such as parent and child.

  • Measure of responsiveness

    – Number of appropriate responses to requests for responses divided by total number of these requests.

❖ Measurements answer the following questions, among others:

  • Are the child's conversations egalitarian, or shared, in nature?

  • Is the child responsive to co-conversationalist(s)?

  • Does the child's ability to demonstrate assertiveness and responsiveness change with different conversation contexts?

❖ Determine how (or if) the child fits into one of the four general patterns of assertiveness and responsiveness.

❖ Select a treatment plan that matches up with this general pattern.

❖ The treatment plan capitalizes on what the child already knows about communication and teaches the child about the communicative process first.

❖ This can be viewed as a functionalist or pragmatic approach to assessment and intervention.

- Children who are active communicators provide themselves with more opportunities to practice language; they already participate in conversations, providing information and responding to their listeners.

  – Their major need is to learn new forms.

  – An expansion of the assertive and responsive acts in their repertoire may be needed.

  – They will tend to incorporate the new forms they learn in their conversations.

  – Clinicians can begin by teaching new forms to fit the old functions already acquired.

- Passive conversationalists first need to develop more assertive conversational acts, both quality and quantity.

  – Once they have increased their use of assertives, new forms can be taught.

  – Clinicians begin by increasing the number and type of assertive acts produced.

- Inactive communicators need to learn to be both assertive and responsive, to participate in conversations, before new forms can be taught.

  – Clinicians need to target these children's contributions to conversations.

  – Nonverbal participation may be a first step.

  – New forms can be incorporated into treatment once some assertives and responsives are produced.

- Verbal noncommunicators need to learn that they must produce conversation bids that are contingent to those produced by their conversation partner(s).

  – Clinicians must increase the child's use of contingent responses.

  – The child must learn to pay attention to the co-conversationalist's utterances.

  – The role of the responder needs to be learned, probably using one example.

  – Once the child has begun to use a limited range of responsive acts, new responsive acts can be taught.

General Language Goals for the 5-Year-Old Child
(Adapted from de Villiers, Roeper, & de Villiers, 1999)

According to these authors, to function communicatively in an age-appropriate manner, and based on recent research findings for preschool-age children, 5-year-olds minimally should demonstrate that they know the following about their first language. Consider the demands that will be placed on the 5-year-old who is about to embark on an academically focused kindergarten program both to demonstrate knowledge and to know how to get the information needed to complete tasks.

- ❖ Pragmatic skills

  - Question-answer mapping, defined as utilizing the right question forms to glean the needed information or action; likewise understanding different question forms to provide appropriate information.

  - Uniquely specifying referents, defined as the child's ability to communicate with sufficient specificity to a listener without the same access to information as the speaker.

  - Linking meaning across referents and events, defined as utilizing elements of cohesive discourse across a number of turns.

  - Point of view, defined as the perspective-taking needed to demonstrate a "theory of mind." That is, the child can take the perspective of the listener, recognizing that there is more than one point of view.

- ❖ In addition, the development of these four features of pragmatics are critical because they interface with the development of deep principles of semantics and syntax.

  - Their data show that normally developing 5-year-olds demonstrate:

    - Wh-word pairing (example: when is related to time)

    - A/the part-whole relationship (example: use of terms anaphorically)

    - Locative-anaphor is present (example: there)

  - The 5-year-old child should be expanding his or her lexicon in terms of its organization as well as increasing its membership both for nouns and verbs.

    - There is more than one name for something, based on specificity: for example, a Toyota, a car, a vehicle.

    - With more words for entities, 5-year-olds become more adept at selecting the best word for a given context.

- ❖ de Villiers, Roeper, and de Villiers (1999) noted that "Language at age five is more than knowing certain words, construction types, and speech acts."

- ❖ They suggest that because language skills at age 5 consist of a close meshing of several essential principles of semantics, syntax, and pragmatics, the assessment procedures that we use to determine sufficient development must reflect this growing sophistication.

- ❖ Thus, the authors note, assessment of these four essential pragmatic features has to reflect the sophistication of the underlying grammar.

INTERVENTION

This subsection includes procedures for providing intervention services to preschool-age children who have been diagnosed with a language disorder, perhaps a Specific Language Impairment, or who have been deemed sufficiently at risk for developing such a disorder during the preschool years. The format of this section will be the same as that for the subsection on assessment.

In this part of the Procedures section, suggestions are made regarding the development and implementation of intervention or treatment strategies with this population. The following topics are covered:

1. General Considerations for Provision of Intervention

2. Intervention Challenges

3. Family-Centered Practices and Programs

4. Where Does Treatment Take Place?

5. Child-Centered Techniques: How Are Focused and General Stimulation Techniques Implemented

6. Specific Child-Directed Speech and Language Techniques

7. Analysis of a Transcript for Child-Directed Speech/Language Techniques

8. Determining Goal Attack Strategies

9. How Do Clinicians Maximize Opportunities for Generalization?

10. Enhancing Treatment Efficacy for Language Disorders

11. Incorporating Early Literacy-Enhancing Activities

12. Implementation of a Phonological Awareness Program (Gillon, 2000, p. 132)

13. How Do We Evaluate the Effectiveness of Our Treatment Programs with Preschoolers?

General Considerations for Provision of Intervention

WHO? These guidelines for intervention should be useful for any speech-language clinician providing intervention services to this population.

WHAT? The general intervention guidelines that follow are relevant for preschool-age children with diagnosed language disorders or individuals who may be older but demonstrating some of the receptive and/or expressive language characteristics of children less than three years of age.

WHY? To provide the most efficacious, that is, effective and efficient, treatment procedures.

HOW? Determine naturalness of approach, and treatment model most appropriate to yield increased communicative competencies.

RESEARCH SUPPORT Compiled from Fey (1986), and Paul (1995).

Clinicians can use this section as a checklist of sorts to be sure that they have thought through the general decisions that have to be made concerning the design of a treatment program. Every client's communication needs are unique in some way, but for all of our young clients we will have to decide where to begin in terms of functional goals, and the role that the clinician will play in terms of service delivery.

❖ Determine whether you will want to use an indirect approach (working through caregivers and others in the child's environment) in a collaborative manner or a direct approach (working directly with the child) or a combination of the two. You may be limited in your choices by rules and regulations imposed by school districts, hospital administrations, and/or third-party payers.

❖ Family-focused treatment is considered a best practice regardless of whether you choose a direct or indirect approach.

❖ Remember that family may mean an extended family group and not a nuclear family unit for a given client. That is, family may include cousins, aunts, uncles, and grandparents. In larger families, older siblings sometimes serve as the young child's most consistent language model and primary caregiver.

❖ Where possible, select treatment approaches that have been shown to have effected change and accelerated progress for children with similar problems; that is, know the latest treatment literature and know the population(s) to which it can be applied.

• Utilize assessment data as a guide in selecting appropriate intervention goals and regimens.

– Remember that you are looking for evidence of the communicative behaviors that are already inconsistently present in the child's repertoire as a place to begin and choosing these prior to other behaviors that have not yet made an appearance. One may serve as a prerequisite for the other.

– Your diagnostic information may also yield evidence of the types of intervention strategies that might work best. For example, was the child likely to imitate you without being asked during the evaluation? Did the child appear to have a higher rate of compliance when you dramatically varied your intonation pattern when making requests? Look for insights that may lead you to make accommodations to the stimuli and instructions you present.

• Periodically reevaluate progress in treatment versus amount of time spent in treatment to determine whether changes in the intervention procedures used need to be made.

• Determine early on whether the family/child share mainstream assumptions regarding role of the caregiver in language learning, use of routine in the home (e.g., dinner time together, a bedtime story read before sleep), and appropriateness of a child as a conversation partner with an adult to avoid later confusion and increase compliance with suggestions made for ways the family can facilitate carryover in the home environment.

• If potential cultural and linguistic barriers to treatment exist, see Goldstein (2000) for suggestions regarding who is most appropriately qualified to provide intervention and how to proceed. See van Kleeck (1994) for suggestions about dealing with cultural mismatching in planning therapy.

• Select goals that are functional for the child's and family's activities of daily living.

• Select goals that will enhance the child's ability to effectively communicate in a variety of settings.

• Be sure that your treatment goals focus on language use and content as well as language form.

• Work collaboratively with other professionals who may be providing services to the child and the child's family.

• Recognize that some families may have other priorities that take precedence over their ability to transport the child to intervention services or consistently follow up with at-home assignments prepared by the clinician.

• Recognize that caregivers are busy people so it will be important to reasonably gauge the amount of time they can spend administering language activities to their child via "homework."

• Recognize that amount of time spent by the caregiver in service of the child's intervention program is not directly correlated with how much the caregiver loves the child or wants to see positive outcomes from therapy for the child.

• Do take information provided by the primary caregivers as credible unless that person or persons has been shown to be an unreliable reporter. In other words, utilize caregivers as much as possible as informants about generalization.

Clinical Insight

We sometimes forget that the family can be our best ally in providing us with information as well as by performing as our surrogates when we are not around. However, these clinicians-in-our-absentia almost always have to receive some training from us so that they can learn what it is that we want them to do. In other words, using parents is not a "freebie"; we have to put in the time to be sure that they understand how to serve as language models or data collectors, for example.

❖ There is support for the efficacy of early intervention. Sometimes we need to convince families and the professionals who refer young children to us that this is so. Ramey and Ramey (1998, pp. 115–118) summarized research on early intervention and found:

- Intervention has greater benefits when it begins earlier and is administered longer.

- When administered more intensively, the outcomes are more positive.

- Direct intervention appears more successful than treatment delivered through training parents only.

- Programs with a broader, more comprehensive focus demonstrate more success than those with a narrower focus.

- There will be individual differences in how children perform following exposure to early intervention services and these differences may be related to the risk factors that qualified the children for the program to begin with.

- If we want children to maintain the gains they have made in early intervention, we either have to structure their environment to support the maintenance of those gains or expect a decrement in those gains.

Intervention Challenges

> **WHO?** These challenges should be addressed by any speech-language pathologist providing treatment services to preschoolers with language disorders.
>
> **WHAT?** These challenges may affect the positive outcomes that can be achieved by any certified speech-language pathologist providing intervention.
>
> **WHY?** Without their consideration, appropriate service delivery cannot be provided.
>
> **HOW?** Consider in turn all of the roadblocks that may prevent changes to communication competencies and brainstorm solutions for them.
>
> **LITERATURE RESOURCES** Compiled from Paul (1995) and others.

If the best offense is a good defense (and I wish I knew who to cite for that pithy statement) in sports as well as life, it also holds for treatment planning for the preschool-age child. Without sounding too pessimistic, think realistically about all of the potential hurdles to progress at the start. Troubleshooting, as we call it, generally turns out to be time well spent.

❖ Duration of the disorder

  • Recognize that language disorders often have a lengthy history and may affect later literacy learning both in the areas of reading and writing.

  • The fact that some language delays do not easily resolve and can become a pervasive part of a child and family's life should be conveyed to families early on.

❖ Literacy enhancing intervention approaches are preferable.

  • There may be a reciprocal, beneficial effect in including goals, targets, and materials that enhance children's awareness and manipulation of both written symbols and the oral representations of those symbols.

❖ Pay close attention to federal guidelines for treatment.

  • Provide therapy within the guidelines of the Individualized Family Service Plan (IFSP) as mandated by federal law:

  • Basic IFSP Information (Fewell, Snyder, Sexton, Bertrand, & Hockless, 1991)

    – What is the child's current status?

    – A description of the family's concerns, their strengths, their needs

    – What are the outcomes expected from intervention?

    – What are the specific intervention services, as yet not provided, that are needed by the child?

    – When will services begin and how long will they last?

    – Who is the specified case manager, responsible for implementing the services?

    – Describe the transition services that are planned for this child.

- Basic IEP Information (Paul, 1995, pp. 332–334)
  - Identifying information about the child and the parents
  - Is this an initial IEP or a follow-up?
  - What is the child's current level of educational performance?
  - What are the child's special education needs?
  - A delineation of annual goals and short-term instructional objectives for meeting those goals
  - What progress has been made toward the goals and objectives delineated? Specify whether the IEP process needs to be continued, modified, or revised with significant alterations.
  - How will accommodations of regular and special education be accomplished to best fit the child's needs?
  - Specify the special services the child will receive in terms of type of service, who will provide it, when and where it will be provided, and the type of service delivery model to be used.
  - How does the child's educational placement comply with the least restrictive environment provision of the Individuals with Disabilities Act?

❖ Enlist familial cooperation. See Pletcher (1995).
  - There are a number of factors that may affect the likelihood of a family's compliance with the intervention program:
    - Their understanding of the necessity for intervention to effect language changes
    - Financial concerns about maintaining long-term treatment
    - Differences in understanding that the family's input is crucial in helping to set goals as well as following through on treatment outside of the clinical setting
    - The need for consistent attendance in treatment
  - The extent of the intra- and extrafamilial network the family can depend on for support in times of health or financial crisis

❖ Serve as a bridge between present family needs and greater independence.
  - Determine how you, the clinician, can best facilitate the family's use of its existing resources and, where necessary to ensure the child's success, help them to identify strategies for meeting unmet needs.

❖ Be clear about your role in the treatment program.
  - Determine whether your role will be that of facilitator or if you will be utilizing induction teaching to effect language growth and change (Olswang & Bain, 1991a).
    - **Facilitation** is a treatment approach that presupposes that the child has the necessary prerequisites for language learning, but that rate of learning can be affected.

- Facilitation speeds up the process or increases the trajectory of learning.
- The child will achieve the same level of competence without treatment, but will not do so as quickly.
- Facilitation brings focused stimulation of input.
- As well as more opportunities for practice and feedback.
- **Induction learning** is a treatment approach teaching new language rules for the understanding and use of new structures, forms, and functions.
- The child's language skills will never achieve the same levels of competence without treatment.
- Induction can be applied whether the child's knowledge of the targeted structure is partial or nonexistent.

Clinical Examples of Facilitation versus Induction Learning

A Clinical Example of Facilitation

Alicia was diagnosed with a language disorder at age 3:4 and enrolled in a mainstreamed preschool classroom where the majority of her classmates appear to be learning language normally. In addition to the language input that Alicia receives from both her teachers and classmates as a result of everyday classroom interaction and the opportunities for her to use language in the course of daily classroom activities, the head teacher in Alicia's room consults with a speech-language clinician who provides suggestions for further facilitating the child's language development.

For example, the SLP suggests that the teachers be sure to bring Alicia together with her classmates who are normal language learners and provide the group of children with guidance in how to specifically interact through conversation. Unfortunately, the SLP explains to the classroom teacher that young children who have problems with language learning are not always included in conversations by their more competent language-using classmates. The teacher needs to guard against interactions that are almost exclusively between teacher and students and rarely between students by assisting children who are more competent with language in finding ways to include children with language disorders.

So, if the teacher finds a group of children playing with the blocks, the SLP notes, suggest that Alicia join in and model some potential dialogue for use among the participants. For example, "Terrance, ask Alicia if you can see what she's building" or "David, I wonder if Alicia knows how to build a ship with blocks. Why don't you find out if she would like to help you?" "That's great, David. Did you notice that Alicia wanted to join your activity but she needed some help from you to figure out how to do it?"

In addition to facilitating interactions between students, the SLP may also help the classroom teachers in focusing on the specific areas of language Alicia finds difficult during her daily activities. If Alicia is having difficulties with plural use, for example, the SLP may show the classroom teacher how to use time spent with Alicia (and her peers) at the sand and water table as an opportunity to address plural formation, by adding appropriate items, for example, cups, spoons, beans, boxes, and so on, in the play routine. If Alicia's difficulties are with asking questions during the classroom's daily group "circle time," then the SLP may suggest some in-class work where the SLP participates in circle time as well, sitting next to Alicia and giving her some suggestions for relevant question-asking.

A Clinical Example of Induction Teaching

Daniel is a 4-year-old with a diagnosed language disorder. Not only is he extremely limited in terms of his use of different sentence structure types and grammatical morphemes, but he does not appear to understand his role in the conversation process. That is, Fey (1986) would probably describe Daniel as an "inactive communicator" because he does not initiate conversation much nor does he more than rarely respond to the conversational bids made by those in his language-learning environment. When he does respond, his responses are often nonverbal in nature. The SLP who works directly with Daniel, and who also serves as a collaborator with his classroom teacher, suggests that Daniel needs to first learn something about the roles and responsibilities of conversation participation before specific linguistic structures will be targeted. Therefore, she begins by working with Daniel on increasing his repertoire of assertive conversation acts (Fey, 1986) like request forms, as well as increasing his consistency of responding to his conversation partners. By using one of Daniel's classmates in a somewhat contrived play interaction, the SLP models simple request forms that are appropriate to the play materials and that are within Daniel's limited expressive repertoire, such as "want Frisbee" or "need more paper," and accompanies these models with actions that elicit the desired responses on the part of the classmate. After the classmate has a turn at requesting using the clinician's models as a base, Daniel is presented with the opportunity to take a turn. With success over time, the SLP adds to the vocabulary used in the requesting activity as well as the degree of difficulty of the request structure used.

Family-Centered Practices and Programs

WHO?   SLPs who want to plan an intervention program to take full advantage of familial involvement.

WHAT?   These programs/procedures focus on and capitalize on the language environment provided by the family.

WHY?   The child spends the most time with family members. It is assumed that the greatest amount and most consistent communicating occurs in this context.

WHEN?   Intervention should always include some family-centered aspects; some programs may call for more direct involvement at different periods of the intervention process.

HOW?   Some specific programs are described in the following. Clinicians must always take family dynamics into consideration when choosing a specific family-centered program.

LITERATURE RESOURCES   See Dunst, Trivette, and Deal (1994); Pletcher (1995).

These family- or caregiver-centered programs are important because, beyond the fact that family involvement is mandated by the federal government, they focus efforts on shaping the behaviors of the child's caregivers to create even more conducive environments for language learning outside the clinical setting. The two references previously listed provide excellent "how-tos" for incorporating parents as collaborators in the intervention process. More specific examples of how family members can facilitate progress in a child's learning about communication competencies follow.

❖ The purpose of family-centered practices is at least twofold:

- To enlist the participation of the child's primary and secondary caregivers so that they feel invested in the child's progress.

- To increase the likelihood of generalization from the clinical setting to the home environment.

❖ Not every family is willing and/or able to participate in a family-centered approach to the benefit of the child at any time or at points during the child's course of intervention.

❖ Without being judgmental, clinicians need to determine the degree to which the family is willing to take on the responsibility of the family-centered approach.

❖ Conducive environments for language learning include: (1) appropriate input, (2) naturalistic contexts for meaningful communication, (3) helpful cuing when necessary, and (4) reasonable expectations for the child's language use. All make it safe for the child to risk success.

- Appropriate input

  - Use language input that conforms to what the child can understand.

  - Generally young children can understand language that is just a bit more complex than the level of their output.

- Naturalistic contexts
  - Help the caregivers to recognize the language-learning potential inherent in activities of daily living.
  - Where they exist, utilize routines for language-learning purposes, for example, bathing, eating, and getting ready for bed.
  - Routines facilitate the mapping of words onto objects and actions because of their repetitive nature, which makes the connection between word and object more transparent.
  - Caregivers will utilize conversations to promote opportunities for the language give and take between themselves and their children.
- Helpful cuing
  - Teach caregivers to increase stimulus support by providing modeling of targets.
  - Caregivers can be shown how to decrease speaking rate to facilitate their child's understanding.
  - Caregivers can be shown how to increase their response latency to make it more likely that their child will participate in conversations.
- Reasonable expectations
  - Provide caregivers with information about the progressive nature of normal language development; that is, language acquisition occurs gradually over time.
  - Foster caregivers' understanding of the specific timelines observed in normal language development.
  - For their child's specific communication needs, promote understanding of necessary prerequisite competencies.
- Risking success
  - Most children with language disorders recognize they have difficulty communicating.
  - When we know we have difficulty doing something, we are less likely to expose ourselves to failure by attempting that something.
  - Help caregivers develop a comfort zone among family members where the child knows that failure is not responded to punitively, but trying your best is encouraged.
- ❖ Most of the already-designed programs focus on conversation as the framework within which to embed new language forms and structures.
- ❖ One general goal of these programs is to teach what for some caregivers is a different approach to interaction with their children.
- ❖ Within conversation this general goal can often be achieved by teaching the caregivers how to:
  - Gauge the length and complexity of linguistic input that their child can comprehend so that appropriate input can be provided.

- Provide a sufficient "response" latency period between the caregiver's turn and the child's turn during conversation exchanges.

- Accept as conversational bids those attempts that are within the child's repertoire; this may mean accepting nonverbal turns.

- Select language goals that are challenging yet targets that can be produced with some success by the child.

Several Programs Currently in Use

❖ These programs have been in use for as many as 20 years, teaching conversation management with children who may be nonverbal and who may have an unknown etiology.

❖ Conversation is viewed as the basis for all communication development; parents are most typically trained for this purpose.

❖ **The Hanen Approach**

- Developed by Ayala Manolson and colleagues.

- Disseminated by The Hanen Centre in Toronto, Canada.

- The Hanen Language Programs include a parent-focused program described in "It Takes Two to Talk": A Parent's Guide to Helping Children Communicate" (Manolson, 1992) and in Girolametto, Greenberg, and Manolson (1986).

- The expressed goals of the Hanen Program are to teach parents the skills needed to be responsive to their children, foster conversational interactions, and provide opportunities for their children to increase their communication skills.

- Training can be completed through workshops offered throughout the year both at the Hanen Centre and in other cities.

- Contact the Centre at: Suite 403, 1075 Bay Street, Toronto, Ontario M5S 2B1, Canada

- (416) 921-1073

- Web site address: www.hanen.org

❖ **The ECO Program**

- Developed by James D. MacDonald and colleagues at Ohio State University.

- Focuses on teaching parents of children who are not yet speaking or who are minimally speaking how to communicate more successfully to enhance language learning (see MacDonald, 1989)

- Development of egalitarian conversations is promoted.

- Parents are taught:

  – Turn-taking skills

  – Observation for signs and signals identified as turns

  – Imitation of child's expressive behaviors is encouraged as acknowledgment of the child's attempts at communication.

❖ **The INREAL Program**

- Originally developed during the 1970s by Rita Weiss and her colleagues at the University of Colorado (Weiss, 1981) and with several updated versions since that time.

- Its name is derived from Inclass REActive Language, promoting intervention in the classroom, that is, opposed to a pull-out model of treatment.

- This treatment approach can be applied to changing the interaction patterns of adults—teachers, SLPs, parents or other caregivers—working with any age population, from toddlers to preschoolers to adolescents to adults with language, learning problems.

- Systematic training focuses on teaching methods for increasing reactivity or responsiveness by "following the child's lead."

- Another important principle is "earning the right" to interact by engaging children in communication activities at appropriate, individualized levels of learning.

❖ **First Steps: Supporting Early Language Development**

- This four-module training program, available in kit form, was published by Educational Productions, Inc., in 1995. The four modules are titled:
  - "Beginning Language Connections"
  - "Reading the Child's Message"
  - "Talking with Young Children"
  - "Building Conversations"

- The program can be used to explain the facilitation of normal language development to parents and other caregivers of children who may be at risk for language-learning difficulties, or as a teaching tool for caregivers of children without any particular language-learning concern.

- The program can easily be used to teach groups of people in an interactive manner.

- The goal of the program is to convey to caregivers the importance of the quality of the linguistic input they provide for the children in their care.

- Each module is comprised of:
  - A videotape describing the principles delineated for each topic
  - A transcript of the videotape segments
  - Prototypes for handouts to be copied for participants
  - A series of suggestions for activities that can be used to enhance understanding of the module's principles and promote discussion among the participants

Where Does Treatment Take Place?

> **WHO?**   Speech-language clinicians providing treatment services to preschoolers.
>
> **WHAT?**   Decisions need to be made concerning the most efficacious contexts for treatment.
>
> **WHY?**   In order to be in compliance with federal mandates, children must receive services in the least restricted environment.
>
> **HOW?**   Systematically explore the pros and cons of options for the contexts of service delivery.
>
> **LITERATURE RESOURCES** See Paul (1995) and Weiss (1997).

The clinician needs to juggle several factors: federal mandates, the child's specific treatment goals, and the available options for treatment. The following factors should be considered:

❖ Historically, several methods of service delivery have been available to SLPs.

❖ Changes in philosophy regarding treatment and subsequent changes in federal legislation have mandated changes in treatment settings.

❖ Treatment should be provided in the least restrictive and most inclusionary environments.

❖ Clinicians need to consider the degree to which the treatment setting itself may facilitate or hinder learning of new concepts and the generalization of those concepts.

❖ The "Pull-Out Model," where the child is removed from his or her typical communication context, is the most restrictive and least inclusionary.

• The child is removed from the preschool classroom and taken to a therapy "room" for intervention.

• Pull-out sessions can be held as individual or group sessions.

• Several of the disadvantages of this approach are:

– Learning is decontextualized so that specific generalization training in a more naturalistic setting will probably become necessary.

– The specific contexts where language is meaningful—in conversation—are typically eliminated.

– Some language targets are best learned and practiced when the child can directly observe their utility in the classroom, for example, requests to the teacher.

– Especially for young children, being taken from their classroom for therapy may be stigmatizing.

• The advantage of this approach is that, for preschool-age children who are easily distracted, the restricted environment may allow for more focus.

– Certain areas of language work, like work on speech sound errors, may be more amenable to "pull out" because of fewer classroom distractions.

– The clinician can more easily provide modeling, monitoring, and feedback with less ambient noise.

- In addition, the other children in the class are not distracted by the child's therapy tasks.

- You can combat the potential stigmatizing effect of therapy by referring to the young child's sessions as his or her "private lessons."

❖ The in-class treatment approach involves provision of intervention in the more natural or usual setting of the preschooler's classroom or, in the absence of preschool, in the child's home.

- One disadvantage of this model:

  - It can be difficult to provide in-class treatment without disrupting the flow of the other children's activities.

- Advantages of this model are:

  - The clinician may be best able to determine the child's specific language needs by observing the demands placed on the child in the classroom.

  - Through observational learning, in-class treatment may also enrich the language learning of the other students in the class.

  - The clinician can use in-class models to teach early literacy skills.

  - Many young children with language disorders are also at risk for difficulties learning to read (see Catts & Kamhi, 1998).

  - Activities that can be focused on to increase a child's language awareness skills include listening and word segmentation abilities.

❖ The collaborative/consultative model may also be used with preschool-age children.

- This usually translates to much less direct service delivery by the clinician than in the other models.

- The clinician may provide collaborative/consultative services to the classroom teacher(s), parents, other caregivers, or other professionals working with the child.

- Consultation time may be spent training others to perform treatment, the selection of appropriate goals for the child based on the observations of the classroom teacher, and the evaluation of the child's progress as a result of the classroom teacher's restructuring of activities in the classroom.

- The advantage of this approach is that:

  - The clinician can more directly utilize the services of the personnel who know the child best on a day-to-day basis.

  - The clinician can spend more time providing services to a larger caseload.

  - The child's "natural habitat" remains largely undisturbed.

- The disadvantage of this approach is that:

  - Some classroom teachers, parents, and special educators feel unqualified to provide these services and believe they have no time to do so.

  - They may also believe that by not providing direct services clinicians are not fulfilling their obligations.

  - The time saved by not providing direct services may be taken up with training others to observe, monitor, and use treatment techniques.

Why Recommend a Preschool or Day Care Placement?

❖ SLPs often recommend that preschool-age children with language disorders be enrolled in some type of group program.

  • Sometimes this recommendation is the only one made following evaluation.

  • Sometimes this recommendation is part of a program that includes some service delivery from the SLP.

❖ The purpose of this enrollment is to increase opportunities for interaction with children and adults in addition to those encountered in the home environment.

❖ Interaction with other children should provide more and varied language stimulation.

  • In a less familiar environment with routines that are different from home, children's language understanding and use are likely to be challenged.

  • Children may need to be more specific because the same knowledge base will not exist between child and teacher as between child and parent.

  • Children may develop code-switching abilities, that is, "school talk" versus "home talk."

  • New vocabulary is likely to be introduced.

  • Additional opportunities for using language for social functions are likely to be introduced.

    – This benefit of classroom placement may not occur naturally and will need some assistance.

    – Remember that children with language disorders are often reticent.

    – Without facilitation by teachers, children with language disorders are likely to be excluded from conversations with normally developing class-mates (Weiss & Nakamura, 1992).

    – SLPs may need to train teachers to watch for this situation.

    – SLPs can demonstrate to teachers methods for including the child with language disorders in conversational interactions with their classmates. These are called "redirects" (Guralnick, 1998).

    – See description of induction teaching previously outlined.

    – Other examples:

      Indirect: "Todd, don't you want to ask Jimmy about that cool front loader he brought to class today? Ask him."
      Direct: "Todd, say, 'Where'd you get that front loader, Jimmy?'" "Say to him, 'How does it work?'"

❖ Preschool programs tend to be more structured and academic in focus than day care programs, thus language learning may be emphasized.

  • Not all placements are equal.

  • There is a great deal of variation between and among preschools and day care settings.

- SLPs should carefully evaluate the curriculum available, ratio of personnel to children, knowledge of personnel about language learning, and so on, before recommending a particular placement.

- Ideally, the program should be language-based in the following ways:

  - All activities should be maximized for their language-learning potential.

  - Classroom personnel should have an appreciation of the value of conversation for normal language learning.

  - Classroom personnel have strategies for including all students in conversation based on their abilities.

  - New, context-sensitive vocabulary should be systematically presented.

  - Opportunities for using new linguistic forms and functions should be available.

  - Materials and activities should be provided that increase the likelihood for discourse development, for example, narratives (storytelling), expository text (explanations), and conversations.

  - Materials also provide the support for memory needed for successful storytelling.

  - Children should be encouraged to participate by "using their words," but nonverbal participation should also be acceptable where appropriate; for example, the child does not have the verbal language easily in his repertoire to participate.

Child-Centered Techniques: How Are Focused and General Stimulation Techniques Implemented?

WHO? SLPs who are providing direct service delivery to children with language disorders or training others to interact in a more language-facilitating manner.

WHAT? Techniques for systematically providing language input that emphasizes language patterns that are focused on the child/client.

WHY? It is important to choose from among the available techniques with a rationale for which technique may be best suited for a child's needs and abilities.

HOW? Steps for implementation of these procedures follow.

LITERATURE RESOURCES Fey (1986), Leonard (1998), Owens (1999), and Weiss (1997).

These are two techniques that are frequently implemented in more naturalistic settings. So, if a child is placed in a "language-based" preschool classroom, presumably all opportunities for enhancing language are taken by teachers and aides. Children may be completely unaware that something special is happening for their benefit.

General Stimulation Techniques

The following factors should be considered:

❖ This is a procedure that provides overall language stimulation to the children exposed to it.

❖ One assumption is that children with language disorders need more exposure to language input.

❖ Another assumption is that the child has been receiving impoverished language input and provision of more input will facilitate the child's catching up with peers.

❖ No specific language goals are delineated for children with a language disorder other than enriching their language-learning environment in all possible ways.

Focused Stimulation Techniques

The following factors should be considered:

❖ Specific goals are selected for children, based on the outcomes of their speech and language evaluations.

❖ Intervention focus is streamlined for the individual child.

❖ The child is bombarded by examples of the targeted form(s) and/or function(s) missing from the child's repertoire.

❖ These examples are presented frequently and in "unambiguous contexts" (Leonard, 1998, p. 197).

❖ Examples may be embedded in natural contexts so that the treatment appears to be more like play and less like drill.

❖ Focused stimulation is a diverse technique:

- It has been used to teach new vocabulary words (Leonard et al., 1982).

- It has been used to teach young children to increase verb complexity (Fey, Cleave, Long, & Hughes, 1993).

❖ Incidental teaching and milieu approach

- These are child-centered approaches and highly naturalistic, thus "ecologically sound" (Owens, 1999, p. 343).

- These techniques can be used in the home, a classroom, or in a clinical environment.

- Select a play situation or utilize the child's activities of daily living to increase the likelihood that the child will attempt to communicate.

- SLPs should follow the child's lead in terms of the child's interests, incorporate appropriate language stimulation, and elicit some relevant production from the child.

- Natural contingencies and reinforcers are utilized, for example, if a child is understood, his or her request can be conveyed and compliance is more likely.

- Warren, McQuarter, and Rogers-Warren (1984) successfully employed the milieu approach in their study that increased children's spontaneous utterance production.

Specific Child-Directed Speech and Language Techniques

WHO?	SLPs can use these techniques in their therapeutic interactions. Parents and other caregivers can also be taught their use.
WHAT?	These are methods of facilitating children's language production that are largely characteristic of mother-child interactions in mainstream families. Clinicians should recognize that these techniques may not be "natural" to persons from all cultures.
WHY?	They vary in terms of the stimulus support provided.
HOW?	Follow the steps outlined in the following. These techniques lend themselves to incorporation into ongoing conversation.

Whenever the term *clinician* is used, parent, teacher, or caregiver could just as easily be substituted as these are techniques that can be easily learned by anyone interacting with young children. As previously intimated in "What?", many parents will tell you that these techniques feel familiar to them, that they already do them. As noted they have been derived from watching "natural" mother-child interactions.

❖ **Imitation**

- The purpose of imitation is to provide a model of correct speech and/or language.

- Use an exact model of what the clinician wants the child to produce.

- Immediate or direct forms of imitation require less processing between hearing the model and producing a replication than delayed forms of imitation that contain a built-in delay in processing time.

  - Examples:

    → Direct Imitation
    Clinician: "Joseph, say, 'I'm ready.'"
    Joseph (age 4): "I'm ready."
    Clinician: "Good job. You said, 'I'm ready.'"

    → Delayed Imitation
    Clinician: "Joseph, say 'I'm ready.' Now you say it, Joseph."
    Joseph: "I'm ready."
    Clinician: "That's right, Joseph. You said, 'I'm ready.'"

- Imitation has been used as the basis of a number of treatment studies with children with language disorders.

- Imitation was particularly popular for use in treatment studies during the time when behavioral models of language learning were the most popular perspective.

- Most frequently, imitation has been used in the teaching of morphological markers or syntactic structures.

  - Mulac and Tomlinson (1977) trained inversion of copula and auxiliary forms.

– Hegde and Gierut (1979) trained nominative case pronouns.

– Gottsleben, Tyack, and Buschini (1974) increased young children's use of basic sentence relationships, for example, subject + verb + object.

- Entire sentences could be trained by breaking them into linear components and then building them up through chaining.

  – Example:

    → Target sentence is "The gorilla is eating the rock."

    → First target "rock."

    → Then, "the rock."

    → Then, "is eating the rock."

    → Then, "The gorilla is eating the rock."

- There are problems with using imitation.

  – It is unnatural; language is usually decontextualized.

  – In treatment approaches utilizing imitation, two- or three-dimensional stimuli have often been added to help provide a context for mapping the imitated form, phrase, and so forth.

❖ Modeling

- The purpose of modeling is to provide the child with examples of appropriate language in particular situations.

- Note in the examples given how repetition is utilized.

- Note how the clinician attempts to make a clear connection between the materials, activities, and the language being used.

- There are several types that are variously related to imitation.

- In parallel talking and self-talk, the clinician's long-term goal may be to increase the child's production of relevant utterances, increase the child's use of a diverse lexicon, or to increase conversational turn length, among others.

  – In parallel talking the clinician talks about what the child is doing. No demand is placed on the child for talking.

  – Example:
  Clinician: "You have the big truck. Yes, you have the big, red truck. I see that you are making the truck go up the ramp. It's going up, up, up the ramp. That big, red truck is going up the ramp."

  – In self-talk clinicians talk about what they are doing, again with no demand placed on the child for speaking.

  – Example:
  Clinician: "I have the red truck. Look! It's going up the ramp. I'm pushing the big truck up the ramp. It's a big truck and I just pushed it up the ramp."

  – Sometimes the clinician will present the child with visual stimuli, for example, pictures, and model a set of descriptions about those pictures.

- After listening to the clinician's models that describe the pictures, the clinician may ask the child to now describe the pictures.

- In this example, the clinician models for the child correct examples of relevant use of is + verb + ing as well as anaphoric use of the pronoun "it."

- Example:
  Clinician: "Here are some pictures I'd like you to look at with me.
  I see a boy riding a bicycle. He is riding it.
  I see a girl mailing a letter. She is mailing it.
  I see a man knitting a sweater. He is knitting it.
  I see a woman hanging a picture. She is hanging it.
  Now it's your turn. Look at my pictures and you tell me about them."

- Sometimes the clinician aids the child in learning the pattern or rule involved in producing a grammatical utterance by presenting the child with some examples that are incorrect, along with those that are incorrect.

  → To accomplish this, the clinician must provide the child with immediate feedback concerning which utterances are correct and which ones are correct.

  → The set of utterances constructed, both correct and incorrect, is referred to as a problem-solving set.

  → Paying close attention to which utterances receive positive feedback and perhaps earn reinforcement and which ones do not, leads to the discrimination of the essential portion of the pattern or rule.

  → As described by Leonard (1981), the problem-solving set may include 25% of utterances that are incorrect as designated as such by the clinician.

- Example:
  Clinician: "I want you to carefully listen to my sentences and see if you can figure out which ones earn points, they're the correct ones, and which ones do not, they're the wrong ones."
  "I see a boy riding a bicycle. He is riding it." Feedback: "That's right."
  "I see a girl mailing letters. She is mailing them." Feedback: "That's right."
  "I see a man knitting a sweater. He is knitting it." Feedback: "That's right."
  "I see a woman hanging pictures. She is hanging it." Feedback: "That's wrong."
  "Now, it's your turn. See if you can figure out how to describe these pictures."

- A variation on this theme is to use what is called a "third person participant."

  → In this approach, another person (perhaps a child) is used to serve as the more competent language user who is able to evaluate the utterances for grammaticality while being observed by the young client.

  → This approach is viewed as closely related to observational learning (Bandura & Harris, 1966).

❖ **Expansion**

- The clinician adds to an utterance produced by the child, thus it is child-centered.

- The clinician's purpose is to produce a correctly formed, adultlike utterance.
- Maintaining the child's topic is essential to this technique.
- The utterance is expanded no farther than the child's original intent.
- Maintenance of both topic and intent is often the clinician's biggest challenges.
- The purpose is to acknowledge the child's attempt but provide an improved version of that attempt.
- Expansion has not been widely used as a treatment technique in the literature.
- One problem may be the inability to reliably determine the child's true underlying meaning.
- Note in the following examples how the clinician attempts to stay within the child's boundaries of intent.
    - Examples:
    Context: Child is observing his dog, Buddy, munching on a large bone.
    Child: "Buddy eat bone."
    Clinician: "Yes, Buddy is eating the bone."
    or
    Context: Child notices that his favorite toy is being played with by a classmate.
    Child: "Teddy play me toy."
    Clinician: "Uh-huh, Teddy is playing with your toy."

❖ **Conversational Recasting/Expatiation**

- Conversational recasting and expatiation are similar to expansion in that the clinician will embellish the child's production to model a correct, adultlike form or structure.
- However, now the clinician extends beyond the child's original topic or intent within a conversational framework.
- The assumption is that this technique not only models more accurate, conventional means for expressing the child's thought, but also provides the child with a suggestion for how to expand the topic within the conversational framework.
- There is less risk of decontextualization because the technique is more naturalistic than imitation, for example.
- The support within a conversation context facilitates the child's ability to map language to the situation and should facilitate generalization.
- Camarata and his colleagues (Camarata & Nelson, 1992; Camarata, Nelson, & Camarata, 1994) have successfully used recasting in teaching expansion of noun and verb phrases.
- Note that in the following examples, a turnabout is provided by the clinician at the end of the recast/expatiation. This is an invitation for the child to take another turn. The turnabout will be italicized.
- The two examples provided have been taken from the previous expansion section, now with recasting applied.

– Examples:
Context: Child is observing his dog, Buddy, munching on a large bone.
Child: "Buddy eat bone."
Clinician: "Yes, Buddy is eating the bone. I wonder what kind of bone it is. *What kind of bone do you think it is?*"
or
Context: Child notices that his favorite toy is being played with by a classmate.
Child: "Teddy play me toy."
Clinician: "Uh-huh, Teddy is playing with your toy. I'll bet he'll be done soon. *Is there something else you can play with?*"

Clinical Insight

Here's something to ponder. If a child with a language disorder has already been exposed to many of these CDTs (Child-Directed Techniques) in the home, that is, if the child's family has been providing him or her with a sufficient quality and quantity of CDTs, why assume that treatment including more of the same will now effect some change? This is a good question and, in fact, there is no reason to assume that children with language disorders learn the same way that children with normally developing language do. We have data to show that sometimes they do not. One way to answer this question and support the use of CDTs is to say that the child was not attending to the input and the clinician's job may be to find ways to make the stimulation more relevant and easier for the purposes of mapping language.

Analysis of a Transcript for Child-Directed Speech/Language Techniques

What to look for:

- ❖ These techniques can be found in combination when typical mainstream play interactions are analyzed.

- ❖ Note how many different techniques have been embedded in this conversation to provide appropriate input for the comprehension levels of the children involved.

- ❖ Note that the input focuses the children on the structures and functions they need to add to their receptive and expressive repertoires to enhance their communicability.

- ❖ Note how these strategies provide opportunities to take turns in the conversation as well as receive appropriate input.

- ❖ By using questions and turnabouts, the clinician automatically provides young children with the opportunity for entering the conversation.

- ❖ Note how many times the clinician or teacher has redirected conversational bids directed to him or her, to another child.

- ❖ Note the degree to which redirection transactions have to be explicitly stated.

- ❖ Remember that we cannot assume that the benefits of normal language modeling will actually occur without some specific direction, at least initially.

Transcript

Context: Max and Jeffrey are interacting with Cindy, a teacher's aide, as they play at the classroom's water table.

Cindy: Max has the biggest measuring cup in the water table [parallel talk]. Well, I think it's the biggest [self-talk]. What do you think, Jeffrey [turnabout]?

Jeffrey: (No response. Jeffrey is fiddling with his shirt.)

Cindy: Doesn't he, Jeffrey [direct, restated request]?

Jeffrey: I think he been playing with water, Cindy.

Cindy: Jeffrey thinks Max has been playing with water [expansion]. Jeffrey, why don't you ask Max what he's been doing with that cup [suggestion to redirect via modeling]? Say, "Max, why are you playing with that cup [imitation]?"

Jeffrey: Max, why you play in the water [attempt at imitation]?

Max: Because I like to.

Cindy: Max says because he likes to [reiteration]. Max, ask Jeffrey what he likes to do [redirect].

Max: Don't want to.

Cindy: Jeffrey looks like he's found something very interesting under the water. Yes! I believe that he has [parallel talking]. Maybe it's a turtle.

Max: That's silly. There's no turtle under there.

Cindy: Hey, don't look at me. Jeffrey's the one exploring. Ask him [explicit redirect].

Max: Jeffrey, do you have a turtle in the water? You don't . . . do you?

Jeffrey: (laughing) No, me no have a turtle. Got a alligator. Rooooooar!

Max: (laughs at Jeffrey's joke) That's pretty silly, Jeffrey.

Cindy: (laughing) You have a pretty good sense of humor, Jeffrey!

Jeffrey: (smiling) Thanks!

Determining Goal Attack Strategies

WHO?   SLPs who have selected speech and language goals as a result of standardized and nonstandardized testing.

WHAT? These represent approaches to the timing of multiple goals in a treatment program.

WHY?   Children's learning style, the nature of the goals themselves, and linguistic strengths as well as needs determine which goal attack strategy will likely be most efficacious.

HOW?   Look at the pros and cons of each of the three goal attack strategies and hypothesize which one best suits your client's temperament and language goals.

LITERATURE RESOURCES Compiled from Fey (1986) and Weiss (1997).

❖ There are at least three different goal attack strategies that can be used.

❖ The *vertical* goal attack strategy:

• One goal is targeted at a time.

• The clinician will target the next goal when the designated criterion level has been achieved.

• Each treatment session focuses on one goal until the criterion level is reached.

• This is one manifestation of the notion, "train deep," where one target receives a lot of attention and presumably is learned very well before moving on.

• Typically, many opportunities for the client to attempt production of the target are planned.

• This is a strategy often associated with a drill mode of treatment (see Shriberg & Kwiatkowski, 1982).

• Who is best served with this strategy?

  – Children who are highly distractible.

  – Children who are beginning work on targets that are not in their repertoires.

  – Children who cannot simultaneously work on multiple targets without becoming confused.

  – Children with very few, and unrelated targets.

  – Example: Child is very immature and has several unrelated targets such as two sounds, /s/ and /g/; and the irregular third-person singular verb form. None of these goals is present in the child's current repertoire.

❖ The *horizontal* goal attack strategy:

• Several goals are targeted within the same session.

- Assumption is that the child can manage to sort out several goals at once (normal language learning works this way; working on one goal at a time wastes time).

- Individual goals are replaced when an individual goal has reached its designated criterion level.

- A new goal can then be selected to replace the one trained to criterion.

- This can be viewed as an example of "train broad," where less time is spent on individual targets per session.

- During the time an individual goal is targeted, however, many opportunities are provided for the client to both receive accurate models and practice production.

- The child is often left to figure out which characteristics, if any, connect the targets together.

- Who is best served by this strategy?

  - Children who are flexible enough to accept frequent changes in goals with maintained attention.

  - Children who are mature enough to recognize that when goals have changed, different patterns of response will be required.

  - Children who have many different language goals to achieve.

  - Example: Child is quite mature and able to pay attention without being prompted by the clinician. This child has several goals that are already inconsistently produced in his repertoire. Mother reports that the child has already begun to generalize to some untrained examples.

❖ The *cyclical* goal attack strategy:

- This strategy is a combination of elements of the vertical and horizontal strategies.

- Assumption is that children learn their language goals by taking what is modeled in therapy and fitting it into their own, internalized, organizational framework.

- A cycle is a designated length of time, such as a semester, a school year, or an 8-week period.

- Assessments are completed to determine the goals prioritized for the first cycle.

- However, within the cycle that is defined by the clinician, several goals are targeted.

- The cycle is divided into individual sessions so that within each of these sessions an individual goal will be targeted.

- Over the course of the cycle, all goals are targeted to some degree; some goals may be targeted for a longer period of time within the cycle than another, depending on severity of the problem.

- Unlike the other two strategies, the emphasis is clearly on modeled input and not on the child's attempts to produce the targets representing the goals.

- Within the cycle the clinician moves to the next goal because it is time to move on; moving is not contingent on progress made toward reaching that goal.

- Reevaluation at the end of the cycle determines which goals need to be retained for a second cycle and which ones have met a preset criterion level.

- New goals can be added for a second cycle to replace those reaching criterion.

- It is expected that generalization to other language goals not specifically targeted will be observed from one cycle to the next.

- It is also expected that rapid generalization will occur to examples of the goal not specifically taught from one cycle to the next.

- Who is best served by this strategy?

  - Children who have multiple goals that are clearly related to one another, for example, multiple phonological processes/patterns, lexical categories.

  - Children who have some evidence of the targeted forms in their repertoire.

  - Children who have demonstrated a tendency to generalize language rules.

A Comparison of Treatment Sessions by Goal Attack Strategies

1. A Session Incorporating a Vertical Goal Attack Strategy for Training the Plural Morpheme /s/, for example, "hats," "packs":

- The child is presented with stimuli to elicit productions of nouns with the plural morpheme /s/. No other goal is targeted during this session.

- A mastery criterion is set (often at 90%).

- Once generalization probes indicate that the child has reached this criterion level, another target is selected. The new target may be production of the plural marker embedded in phrases or sentences.

- Or, the next target may be another phonetic form of the plural marker, /z/, for example, "crabs," "designs."

2. A Session Incorporating a Horizontal Goal Attack Strategy for Training the Plural Morpheme /s/, for example, "hats," "packs."

- The child is presented with several goals within the same session so time for the session is divided among the goals.

- Each goal is assigned a criterion performance mastery level.

- Perhaps all three phonetic variations of the plural morpheme are targeted within one session, but as separate goals, that is, /s/, /z/, and /iz/, for example, "matches," "bunches."

- Or, the clinician may target several other morphemes unrelated to the plural marker within the session. For example, article use, or politeness, or irregular past tense, may also share time with plurals during treatment.

- Once the mastery level has been reached for any of the goals in generalization probes, a new goal replaces the old.

3. A Session Incorporating a Cyclical Goal Attack Strategy for Training the Plural Morpheme /s/, for example, "hats," "packs."

- Although a number of different speech and language goals may be targeted during the cycle, only one goal, perhaps /s/, is attacked per session.

- Once the designated length of time for goal targeting has been completed, for example, four sessions, the next goal is targeted, regardless of progress made or lack thereof.

- Reevaluation of all goals is completed at the end of the cycle to see which goals should continue to be addressed and which ones are no longer viable.

- Typically, closely related goals work best using this strategy. For this child, the three phonetic variations of plurals, possessives, and third-person singular verb forms, might all be targeted within a single cycle, but not more than one per session.

How Do Clinicians Maximize Opportunities for Generalization?

WHO?	All SLPs who are providing intervention should be concerned about their client's generalization to untrained examples.
WHAT?	Generalization refers to the ability to learn underlying rules or patterns that allow the child to generate novel instances of a trained structure, for example.
WHY?	Generalization is essential to demonstrating the success of therapy; dismissal from therapy may rely on whether or not the child can generalize.
HOW?	See the procedures outlined in Hughes (1985) for making accommodations to the treatment context and the home environment to facilitate generalization learning.

The name of the clinical "game" is generalization. Without it, we are not successful clinicians. Since we cannot hope to teach every example, we have to teach a representative subset in such a way that the child can generalize what has been learned from a relatively small number of examples to the whole class of possibilities. This is not a small order. Here are some definitions of two generalization types and suggestions for how to go about this major task.

❖ For children to be successful language learners, they have to succeed at both stimulus generalization and response generalization.

- Stimulus generalization refers to generalization across settings. For example:

  - From the therapy room to the classroom

  - From the classroom to the playground

  - From conversation with the clinician to conversation with a parent

  - From conversation with the clinician from one semester to the next clinician assigned to the case

  - From the classroom to the home environment

  - From use of stimulus cards to use in conversation

  - Example:
    Ashley's clinician is targeting an increase in the child's use of appropriate responses to When? questions using a storybook called *Barry's Big Day*. This book lends itself to the asking and answering of When? questions. The clinician suggests that Ashley's teacher may want to use the same book during a classroom activity where all of the children, including Ashley, can participate in responding appropriately to When? questions. Ashley demonstrates that he can generalize his appropriate responses to When? questions to both the classroom teacher and to a group book-reading setting.

- Response generalization refers to generalization to new examples not specifically trained in therapy. For example:

  - From teaching examples at the single-word level to other untrained examples at this level

– From trained examples in initial word position to untrained examples in final word position

– From trained examples at the single-word level to production of untrained examples at the multiword level

– From trained examples at the multiword level to the conversation level

– From trained examples of copular "is" to examples of auxiliary "is"

– Example:
Ashley's clinician has been targeting Ashley's use of the regular plural morpheme in single words in response to cards depicting either one item or multiple examples of the same item, for example, "marble," "marbles." Now the clinician divides the cards between them and models, "I have marbles and cookies. What do you have?" Ashley responds with "I have toys and elephants." This indicates that Ashley has generalized his plural use to a more sophisticated linguistic level.

❖ Hughes (1985) suggests two basic approaches to facilitate generalization between the therapy environment and the home environment:

• Make the clinical setting more like the home environment. For example:

– Have the child bring toys, books, or other materials from home.

– Use the primary caregiver from home as part-time therapist in the therapy setting.

– Emphasize that the two settings are not completely different. That is, language learned in the clinic is useful for communication at home and vice versa.

• Make the home environment more like the clinical setting.

– Have the child take therapy cards and other stimuli from the therapy setting home for structured or unstructured interactions.

– Have the primary caregiver use a therapy regimen in the home setting.

– Emphasize that the two settings are not completely different. That is, language learned at home is useful for communication in the clinic and vice versa.

❖ Provide a variety of examples that allow the child to learn the breadth of the language rule or pattern.

• Train "deep" is a good technique for establishing a new language form or function.

– Lots of examples of very similar stimuli

– Probably deal with only one or two different goals at a time

• Train "broad" is a good technique for expanding the specific examples trained into the learning of a more general rule.

– Utilize examples that are more and more dissimilar from one another

– Vary settings and contexts to prompt the child's need to figure out why these stimuli belong to the same "set"

❖ An example of teaching English plurals via "train deep"

- Child has no evidence of plurals in his or her repertoire

- Provide examples of similarly formed plurals

❖ Select representative examples that should help the child observe the topographical similarities among the set of examples.

❖ There should be enough variation in the examples to allow the child to form an appropriate response set.

- To teach the concept of regular plural formation in English, you probably need to provide examples of all three plural forms.

- Provision of only one of the morphophonemic variants, such as "hats," might be too narrow to form the complete response set, for example, "matches," "pools."

❖ Be sure that the examples are functional; if they are useful in activities of daily living, they are more likely to be used and to transfer to other settings.

- For example, see Olswang, Kriegsman, and Mastergeorge (1982) for systematic training of requesting across settings.

Enhancing Treatment Efficacy for Language Disorders

WHO? Any SLPs who are providing intervention for children with language disorders.

WHAT? We need to know whether the intervention services provided are effective and efficient. Are children making faster progress and more qualitative gains than they would without therapy?

WHY? We have to be able to justify the expense and time for therapy.

HOW? See Olswang and Bain (1991) and Campbell and Bain (1991) for specific procedures and measures of efficacy.

Clinical Insight

The American Speech-Hearing-Language Association is supporting the collection of treatment outcomes data nationwide with one of the targeted populations being preschool-age children with language disorders. We know that virtually all of the approaches attempted with young children with language disorders have worked at least some of the time for some children. What we need to know is which treatment approaches are most likely to work best with which children to create better client-approach matches.

It is important that we use the treatment data available to us in the literature to make decisions about what works and what does not via treatment. Most of the data we have are in the form of group subject designs, single-subject designs, and case studies.

❖ Determining efficacy is sometimes difficult because treatment outcomes are often reported as group data. Thus, it is unlikely that each participant equally contributed to the positive treatment effect.

❖ Single-subject designs allow clinicians to more clearly observe an individual subject's changes over time.

❖ A number of studies have compared two or more treatment approaches to look for differential effects on their child subjects.

• Differences in cognitive abilities

• Differences in the specific behaviors being targeted

• Differences in other individual characteristics. For example, is the language form present in the child's repertoire?

❖ Some important research findings with regard to imitation:

• Imitation approaches may be superior to more naturalistic approaches, for example, incidental teaching.

• Imitation requires production practice and incidental teaching does not.

• If you are trying to establish new language structures in a child's productive repertoire, imitation may provide some early success.

❖ Some important research findings with regard to modeling:

- Studies have compared modeling approaches that provided production practice and those that did not.

- Ellis Weismer and Murray-Branch (1989) found superior performance when children had production practice.

- Rate of input can also be an important variable; children with language disorders may perform better when the input they receive is slower than what can be easily handled by a normally developing child.

❖ Some important research findings with regard to recasting:

- A comparison of recasting and imitation demonstrated a decided advantage for conversational recasting (Camarata, Nelson, & Camarata, 1994).

- Leonard (1998) suggests that this is counterintuitive because recasting does not require production practice but imitation does.

- Conversational recasting may work well because it is:
  - Highly contextualized
  - Child-centered
  - May foster motivation

❖ Some important research findings with regard to parents as clinicians:

- Fey, Cleave, Long, and Hughes (1993) compared clinicians and parents providing treatment.

- Both groups of subjects made progress; more consistent gains were made by children receiving treatment from SLPs.

❖ Some important research findings with regard to pretherapy skill levels:

- Post-hoc testing of children with SLI assigned to different treatment groups.

- Children with lower aptitude scores were more successful with imitation approaches.

- Children with higher aptitude performed better with more naturalistic approaches, for example, focused stimulation and incidental teaching.

Incorporating Early Literacy-Enhancing Activities

WHO? SLPs who are interested in helping children bridge the learning of oral language and reading and writing.

WHAT? Some activities can focus children on the aspects of language that may enhance literacy learning such as phonological awareness and inferencing.

WHY? Research has shown that there is a positive correlation between children's oral language skills and the likelihood that they will learn to read and write at a normal rate.

WHEN? These activities can be incorporated throughout intervention programming.

HOW? Procedures for incorporating early literacy-enhancing activities follow.

RESEARCH SUPPORT See Catts and Kamhi (1998), Gillon (2000), van Kleeck, Gillam, and McFadden (1998) for research support.

Given what we know about the close connection between children's success in learning to read and having age-appropriate language skills as a base, it seems intuitive that we would want to be sure to do whatever we can to assist the child who already demonstrates difficulty with language learning (oral language skills) to make the transition to decoding written language symbols. One way to do this is by emphasizing language competencies that researchers have shown are prerequisites to literacy learning.

❖ Never underestimate the incorporation of text into treatment materials.

• Written symbols may serve as additional cuing for children trying to decipher messages.

❖ Even when the clinician does all of the reading, children are exposed to the wonderment of text when information is conveyed in this medium.

• Research shows that exposure to text in any form, such as refrigerator notes, recipes, newspapers, and observing caregivers reading, increases children's curiosity about text and figuring out how to decipher the code.

• Some early sound-symbol relationships can be fostered and may serve to cue the child to the whole answer you are looking for.

❖ Consider using written labels for items, especially new vocabulary words that you are targeting, even when you have no expectation that the child can read them.

• The child may eventually glean the sound-symbol relationship from this juxtaposition.

❖ Use storytelling, story retelling, or any other type of narrative-based treatment process where appropriate and feasible as the basis for at least some of your treatment.

• Narrative structures are frequently used as the basis of language learning in mainstream curricula.

- Children who have been frequently read to have been shown to have learned about story grammar, which allows them to anticipate the type of information that will be provided in the story and permits them to inference with more success.

- When children learn story grammar conventions, they develop a template that assists them in developing their own stories (writing or telling) as well as deciphering the stories of others (reading or listening).

- See Stein and Glenn (1979) for a description of story grammar component parts.

- The learning of story grammar also aids children in language perspective taking.

- For example, ask children if something is missing in their understanding of a story.

- For example, when children create a story with your help, ask them what information has to be included so that new listeners or readers will be able to understand the story.

❖ Encourage children to speculate about what might happen next when using process/experiential activities.

- For example, use the making of popcorn as the basis of an activity targeting new vocabulary and new syntactic structures. Ask: "What do you think will happen if we put in too much oil?" Or, "Uh-oh. Our popcorn popper isn't working. What could be the problem?"

Implementation of a Phonological Awareness Program
(Gillon, 2000, p. 132)

❖ Research has shown that a direct approach to teaching literacy is more effective than an indirect approach.

❖ If a child demonstrates severe deficiencies in the area of phonological awareness, it may be necessary to implement an intensive model of treatment, either for individuals or small groups.

❖ Focus on developing phonemic level skills within a phonological awareness framework.

❖ Integrate phonological awareness activities with the training of letter-sound correlations.

❖ Instruction in phonological awareness will be most efficacious after the child has had some general language instruction.

❖ Be sure to incorporate a range of activities that focus on phonemic analysis and synthesis activities.

❖ Be sure to include activities that involve phoneme segmentation skills.

❖ Activities selected should engage the child to reflect on how the phonological system is organized; use manipulative materials to help with this engagement on the part of the child.

How Do We Evaluate the Effectiveness of Our Treatment Programs with Preschoolers?

WHO? SLPs who must maintain accountability for the treatment they provide.

WHAT? The measurement of change in our preschool-age client's communicative behaviors following administration of a therapy program.

WHY? Two reasons: (1) to demonstrate accountability and (2) to make changes in the treatment plan to increase its efficacy.

HOW? A procedure to troubleshoot our treatment program follows.

LITERATURE RESOURCES See Fey and Cleave (1990) and Olswang and Bain (1994).

This is one of those topics that could have been placed as easily in the Assessment portion of this section as in the Intervention portion. One of the primary functions of evaluation procedures is to allow us to periodically assess the changes our clients have made over time. These important data will let us know if sufficient progress has been made and, if not, where we can look to make changes in the programming.

❖ To evaluate the progress made as a result of a treatment program designed for young children, we have to be sure that we are evaluating the effects of the *program* and not the effects of maturation.

❖ Plan treatment in such a way that baseline data are collected early to serve as a comparison for later performances. Collect baseline data on several language behaviors that will not specifically be targeted in treatment. Fey and Cleave (1990) call these "control goals."

❖ Perform periodic evaluation of your young client's progress. Probably after a month's time in treatment (unless you have only seen your client twice in that time), institution of some form of treatment evaluation should be undertaken.

Clinical Insight

Clinicians disagree about how soon after the institution of treatment this should be done. I think that this decision often is made based on a number of factors, including the intensity of the particular child's treatment program, the dictates of the school or center for which you work, the dictates of third-party payers, and your clinical intuition. Most seasoned clinicians get a good "feel" for whether the child is struggling with the goals and treatment plan as designed.

• Select representative language behaviors for testing that have not been specifically trained in the treatment program although they are related to those that have been (these represent generalization goals) and those that have been directly targeted.

• Obviously, if your treatment plan is working well for your client, you should see it reflected in high levels of accurate performance on the target goals and some evidence of progress on the generalization goals selected.

- What you do not expect to see is progress on the "control" goals because these presumably bear no relationship to the targeted goals. If you do, then Fey and Cleave (1990) suggest that you question the role of maturation in the child's demonstration of progress. If maturation has played a part, then to what extent was your treatment necessary?

❖ In addition to looking for evidence of specific gains on targeted, generalized, or control goals, we need to think about progress more ecologically. That is, has the child made gains that positively affect his or her ability to function in the world?

- This is also an issue of the social validation of treatment. How has the treatment plan affected the child's ability to communicate in his or her world?

  – How do the child's parents and other caregivers view progress made? Ask family members if the child is now able to meet communication demands in the home environment in ways not evident prior to treatment.

  – How do classroom teachers and related personnel view progress made? Ask the school personnel if the child is now able to meet communication demands in the school environment in ways not evident prior to treatment.

  – How does the child view the progress? Ask the child, if the child has appeared cognizant of having communication difficulties, if she or he has found communicating easier, less anxiety-provoking perhaps, than prior to the start of therapy.

❖ If the child has made little or no progress, look at the following parameters of the treatment plan and consider changes:

- Amount and type of stimulus support provided: Is there enough? Are the types of prompting and cuing provided sufficient and meaningful to the child?

- Are enough examples being provided and arranged in such a way to make obvious the language rule that is being targeted?

- Are the goals selected and the examples being taught functional for the child? That is, are they inherently motivating?

- Is sufficient response latency being provided? Perhaps the child needs additional time to process responses as well as the stimulus support being presented.

- Explicitness or implicitness of feedback provided: Is it explicit and consistent enough? Does the child always know when he or she has provided a correct response so that the basis for self-correction and self-monitoring is being developed?

- Type of response expected from the child: Is the response so far out of the child's repertoire that the child cannot possibly comply? That is, the clinician may have miscalculated and prerequisites of the response are not part of the child's repertoire.

- Is the child's program focusing on treatment that is too deep or too broad in nature, so that the child cannot get the "big picture" from which to generalize?

- What else is going on in the child's life that may be negatively impacting the ability to make progress in treatment, perhaps illness, family disturbance, or depression, and can any of these factors be modified?

- Does the child need a break from treatment? Perhaps the child and/or others in the child's family believe that the child has made sufficient progress and no longer see the utility for treatment.

❖ Dismissal decisions are sometimes made when no progress in treatment has been observed despite both minor and major changes in the treatment focus. According to Fey (1988), decisions to dismiss a child from therapy should never be considered irrevocable but rather decisions that are appropriate at that point in time.

SECTION

CASE STUDIES

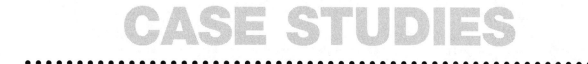

CASE 1: "LATE TALKER" WITH PROBABLE DIAGNOSIS OF SLI

Child: 3-year, 6-month-old male named "Tony"

Referral Source and Concerns: Both of the child's parents and the child's physician expressed concern about Tony's delayed development of language. The parents called to make the evaluation appointment and requested the first available appointment time. The child's pediatrician stated in her referral letter that her repeated suggestions over the last 2 years to the parents to have Tony evaluated were not followed up. The child's day care classroom teacher has also been requesting that the parents have the child evaluated. The teacher's concern, however, was centered on Tony's poor social and behavioral skills; she believed that she could no longer control him in the classroom.

Background: Tony is the only child of an upper middle-class white, married couple. Both parents are employed outside the home. Mother accompanied the child to the evaluation and served as the informant. Tony has a history of recurrent middle ear infections with the first diagnosed around 6 months of age, delayed language expressive development (about 100 intelligible words, some two- and three-word combinations), and precocious motor development, all documented by the pediatrician's referral letter. When the mother called to request an evaluation appointment, she had described her son as a "busy boy" who always seems to have "his own agenda" that makes it difficult to get him to do an activity other than one he initiates.

Step 1: Preassessment

I called the family prior to the evaluation date and explained the general "flow" of the evaluation. Tony's mother answered the phone and she acknowledged that she and her husband still thought that Tony was a normal child, albeit "learning language his own way." They had decided, however, that they would go through with the evaluation just to officially rule out the presence of a problem. I explained the approximate length of the evaluation, asked whether the child will be at his peak performance level at the time of the late-morning evaluation, for instance, too close to nap time? meal time? and asked what I could do to ensure the child's best cooperation. I suggested that the parent, or whoever will be accompanying the child, bring along a toy and/or book that the child is particularly fond of. I also asked what types of materials the child prefers to play with: Are books meaningful? Does the child like to draw or paste? I also told the parent that she may be asked to participate in portions of the evaluation.

I asked the parent what her family's goal(s) was for the evaluation. That is, what questions did they want to have answered? We discussed the kinds of information that the family could expect to gain by the end of the evaluation session, for example, whether or not a diagnosis of a language disorder could be made, recommendations for treatment given, explanation of etiology, and so on. I assured the mother that my goal was to provide the family with my professional opinion by the end of the evaluation about the appropriateness of Tony's speech and language development as compared with his peers. I would also hope to be able to provide some suggestions for how to proceed if a language disorder was diagnosed.

Step 2: Assess Child

My priorities were the following:

- Rule out hearing loss and intellectual deficit either through my own testing or via referral to other professionals (e.g., audiologist, clinical psychologist).

- At the time of the evaluation have the mother and her son interact for 10 to 15 minutes, with the clinician in a separate observation room where possible, to investigate the communicative demands placed on the child by the parent and how the child responds to these demands. A portion of the language sample can be collected during this time as well, but a more complete language sample will be collected to determine whether the child is combining words and, if so, the extent of the child's repertoire of semantic relationships.

- The only standardized test directly administered to the child was the *PPVT-III* (Dunn & Dunn, 1997). This choice was made because of the issues of vocabulary development and the desire to corroborate the mother's impressions of her son's expressive vocabulary with a standardized test of receptive vocabulary.

- During testing by the clinician, the mother was asked to complete the MacArthur Communicative Development Inventory (Fenson et al., 1993) to obtain a standardized measure of the child's vocabulary development.

- Formal and informal evaluation procedures should yield information about the manner in which the parent(s) interact with their son, the opportunities they provide for him to use the language he does have, as well as the language demands they place on him in terms of both the level of language input they provide and the quality of output they expect.

- It will be important to note, too, which communicative intentions the child uses either verbally or nonverbally, or with a combination of symbols.

Results of Testing:

Following a hearing screening that revealed adequate hearing for purposes of speech and language learning on this particular day, Tony and his mother interacted for approximately 10 minutes playing with a variety of toys in an observable treatment room. The clinician noted that Tony rarely initiated any interactions with his mother either verbally or nonverbally via gesture, but that he would respond, usually nonverbally, to her requests for actions, attention, or objects. Rarely did the mother make any requests for information from her son that could not be conveyed nonverbally.

The child did not transition easily from interacting with his mother to working with the clinician. Once the clinician was finally able to take over without the constant presence of the mother, the mother began to complete the vocabulary checklist. Tony appeared to have little interest in the pictures the clinician showed him that were part of the standardized test materials (*PPVT-III*, for example) so the clinician resorted to nonstandardized assessment, using objects for evaluating semantic relationships and comprehension of some of Brown's 14 Grammatical Morphemes, such as "Show me shoes" comprehension of the plural morpheme and asking him to tell me "What's that?" when showing him the figure of a man riding a horse (i.e., if he says "ride horse" or "man horse" this may indicate semantic relations usage), as well as single-word vocabulary.

The language sample collected over the course of the hour-long evaluation yielded data that demonstrated an MLU of 1.32, falling more than two standard deviations below the mean for Tony's age of 42 months. There were only two examples of Brown's 14 Grammatical Morphemes: a production of the preposition "in" and one of the plural form ("cookies"). Tony appeared to be a child who fell into Fey's (1986) category of "passive conversationalist," one who recognizes his need to be responsive but is unaware or typically unable to fulfill the role of communication initiator. A very limited set of communicative intentions were noted. Similarly, the child's vocabulary as per the mother's completion of the MacArthur Communicative Development Inventory and corroborated by the language sample analysis, revealed an immature expressive vocabulary. Tony was mostly intelligible when producing the few single words he did produce during the evaluation. It was noticeable, however, that when he combined words, he became less easily understood.

Step 3: Provide Diagnosis and Recommendations

My diagnosis of a significant speech and language disorder that could be characterized as SLI was made on the basis of the data collected during this evaluation by both the clinician and the mother (MCI). I explained to the mother that none of the areas of Tony's language that were evaluated were functioning close to the normal range of performance expected for a child 42 months of age. I also explained something about the term *SLI* and showed her how Tony's history as a "late talker" may have been a warning that he was at greater risk to persist in his language disorder and earn the label of SLI. We also talked about the course of this disorder and particular factors of concern, that is, Tony has both receptive and expressive deficits. The mother began to cry at hearing the news, but after a few minutes said she had known there was a problem but could not face it until recently.

I then made recommendations for speech and language intervention to begin as soon as possible to attempt to facilitate an increase in Tony's overall language abilities, both in terms of his language comprehension and speech and language expression. Options for service delivery were also provided. Specific treatment recommendations were delineated as follows:

- An SLP should provide Tony's parents with information about expectations for normal speech and language development in preschool-age children so that they will fully understand the scope of Tony's speech and language delays. They should be counseled about the best ways to encourage Tony to use his new language skills in the classroom (see the next recommendation) and at home with other co-conversationalists.

- Given the options available in his school district, Tony should be enrolled in a half-day classroom program designed for preschoolers with significant communication disorders. This setting will provide ongoing monitoring of Tony's progress as well as ongoing structured, facilitated opportunities for his conversation interactions with his classmates.

- When Tony has become more acclimated to classroom intervention procedures, some one-on-one intervention may be tried specifically to work on improving the precision of his articulation in connected speech and for learning new forms, for example, to use word categories not yet present in the child's repertoire, to increase his repertoire of semantic relationships, and to facilitate the emergence of grammatical morphemes.

- A general increase in the frequency of Tony's linguistic output, especially to initiate topics or make other assertive conversation bids such as statements, comments, and requests for information, should also be targeted by his clinician. Fey's (1986) program for work with children who are "passive conversationalists" should be considered as an eventual framework for therapy. This was explained to the mother.

- I suggested that Tony be reevaluated in 6 months to see if there was evidence that the program was providing the child with greater benefits than we would have expected to have seen in 6 months of time by maturation alone.

Step 4: Intervention

- The classroom setting recommended provided Tony with a generalized stimulation type of intervention. That is, he was bombarded with modeled language input at appropriate levels of complexity for his comprehension level, and language routines that all of his classmates participated in such as talking about the calendar, the weather, planning their day, and group activities based on a story the class focused on for the week.

- The SLP was able to see Tony twice weekly for 30 minutes, once alone outside of the classroom to work on increasing his intelligibility and once for 30 minutes inside the classroom where she worked at fostering his use of assertives in interactions with other classmates and his teacher. This also gave the clinician the opportunity to model for the classroom teacher and aides how to help Tony participate more fully in conversational turn taking with his classmates and giving him the frequent opportunities to do so.

- The SLP also met with Tony's parents once per month in their home for the first 6 months after the child was enrolled in the classroom program and individual treatment to discuss their son's speech and language behaviors as they observed them at home and to suggest ways to carry over what was learned in therapy to the home environment. These meetings lasted about a half hour and were scheduled, when possible, at times when both mother and father could attend.

Step 5: Outcomes of Intervention

- Although Tony was initially reticent and withdrawn in the classroom, he slowly became comfortable with the play as well as with the more academic routines and was encouraged to participate by his teachers at levels that were within his repertoire of responding.

- It was necessary for his teachers to do a great deal of modeling to show him how he could use language to facilitate his interactions with his classmates. After about a month, he had begun to say "hello" spontaneously to other children and adults when he entered the room in the morning and said "bye" to them when leaving.

- Tony's parents reported that their son was generally using a lot more language at home, was attempting new words on a daily basis although they have not yet heard any of the inflectional morphemes that have been targeted. His behavior had also improved, especially since transitioning from one activity to the next had become less traumatic for him. Moreover, the child expressed his eagerness to attend school every morning and was disappointed when Saturday morning was a "no school?" morning.

- The parents noted that, although they had formerly used a great deal of verbal praise to reinforce Tony's verbal attempts, they now noticed that communication seemed to have become its own reward for Tony. That is, once he discovered that a word or phrase "worked" for him, for instance, "want cookie," he was very happy to repeat it at different times and in different contexts.

- The clinician who was monitoring his case was not yet convinced that Tony was benefitting from one-on-one sessions outside of the classroom to work on speech sound productions. Because his needs appeared to be so much more basic communicatively, she suggested that Tony receive both of his 30-minute sessions in the classroom.

- A follow-up appointment at our clinic revealed that the child had blossomed in terms of language learning. Although he remained delayed in both his language comprehension and production, his test scores revealed more than 12 months worth of gains in the 6 months since we had seen him, providing evidence for an efficacious program.

CASE 2: PRESENCE OF A PRESCHOOL LANGUAGE DISORDER WITH SLI LIKELY

Child: A 5-year, 2-month-old female child named "Emily"

Referral Source We received a referral to evaluate Emily on the recommendation of her kindergarten classroom
and Concerns: teacher who was concerned that the child was not able to keep up with her classmates on any
activities involving storytelling. Emily had first drawn the teacher's attention because she was a very
quiet child. Emily's mother agreed to have her daughter evaluated, noting that "language isn't her
strongest area, but she does everything else real well."

Step 1: Preassessment

Once a date for her daughter's evaluation had been scheduled, I called Emily's mother at work and asked her to describe Emily's speech and language abilities to me. The mother noted that Emily had not been precocious like her older sister, Joan, but the mother knew that second children did not usually talk as early or as much as older siblings and anyway, children are all so different she did not see why she should expect both girls to be the same in their development. All of Emily's language milestones appeared to have occurred roughly on time, as did her developmental milestones in motor and social-emotional development, according to Emily's mother's report. In addition, Emily was a very smart child, in her mother's opinion, able to learn how to work a new computer program with little or no instruction. The child preferred playing alone but got along very well with other children when she did play in groups. Her mother was aware that some of the children in the neighborhood had initially teased Emily because of her quiet ways, but now they had gotten so used to her that they seemed to have accommodated her limitations by just asking her fewer questions. When Emily started school, her mother claimed to have been somewhat apprehensive that her daughter would have a difficult time keeping up with her classmates, but she figured her daughter would do with them what she had always done at home: use gestures and highly communicative if limited utterances to get her point across. No history of hearing loss or a history of episodes of middle ear disease was reported. Emily was described as a well-adjusted, happy child, but her mother claimed that her daughter did have some idea that she could not talk like the other kids and that she was sometimes embarrassed by this.

Emily's classroom teacher, with the permission of the child's mother, sent a letter chronicling her concerns about Emily. She described the child as well-adjusted and well-behaved, who participated willingly in group activities although her ability to contribute verbally was limited relative to her peers. The teacher also described Emily's attempts at sentences as sounding very immature, with most of the word "endings" left off. Sometimes this made Emily difficult to understand and requests for clarification from the teacher and Emily's classmates were not uncommon. Emily was always willing to try to clarify but often resorted to gestures to do so.

Step 2: Assess Child

My priorities were the following:

* Rule out hearing loss and intellectual deficit either through my own testing or via referral to other professionals (e.g., audiologist, clinical psychologist). Although I have no reason to suspect hearing loss, given the child's history, it is critical to test the hearing of any child brought to you when the concern is language development.

* Complete a comprehensive test of language competencies. I chose the *PLS-3* because I wanted both a measure of receptive language and a measure of expressive language.

* I chose to collect a language sample, divided into several portions, one where the child's mother was an interactant, one where I was (an interactant unfamiliar to the child), and for the last portion Emily talked with Doris, Emily's best friend, who was able to accompany Emily to the evaluation. I wanted to see how consistent the quantity and quality of Emily's speech and language were across different interactants. I also planned to use this sample to calculate several pragmatic, lexical, and syntactic/morphology measures, for example, assertiveness and responsiveness ratios, type-token ratio, and MLU and DSS (using a computer program for both).

* I administered the *PPVT-III* (Dunn & Dunn, 1997) not only because it yields a receptive vocabulary age but because of the high correlation between this score and IQ measures. This will provide a very gross measure of Emily's intellectual ability.

* Although no concerns about Emily's intelligibility had been expressed, I planned to complete a separate articulation test just to substantiate that she had all of the sounds in her sound repertoire that were necessary for production of the grammatical morphemes. The language sample data were used to cross-check the single-word data collected so that a more comprehensive picture of Emily's intelligibility could be formed.

- I wanted to evaluate Emily's stimulability for production of the grammatical morphemes she spontaneously omitted so I prepared a probe list of grammatical morphemes in phrases and sentences and put together a set of pictures that I believed would elicit production of these morphemes, for example, possessive marker.

Results of Testing:

As expected, the hearing test demonstrated normal hearing acuity bilaterally. Emily was easily trained to raise her hand in response to hearing the sound presented under headphones.

Emily willingly completed all of the tests presented to her. The test battery, including the collection of language samples, lasted approximately 90 minutes. Emily was less willing to engage me in conversation than she was her mother and friend. Although I tried very hard to use only open-ended questions and comments to encourage her participation, I probably used more limiting questions to get some responses from her than I would have liked to have done.

The results of the standardized testing revealed a picture of an expressive-only language problem. Both the receptive portion of the *PLS-3* and the *PPVT-III* yielded scores well within normal limits for Emily's chronological age. In fact, her receptive vocabulary age was almost one year higher than her chronological age. Her language sample, on the other hand, revealed almost total omission of inflectional verb markers; at no time did Emily produce anything but a present tense verb. This resulted in a DSS score that was several years below her chronological age; no sentences earned sentence points and the main verb category was filled with many attempt markers but few other credits. The probe list that I had prepared also bore this out. When asked to imitate my productions of picture description, Emily was capable of producing the morpheme in question but without my model she consistently left off the targeted ending. Her completion of the articulation test was unremarkable in its findings; Emily was able to produce all of the sounds of English with apparent ease.

Step 3: Provide Diagnosis and Recommendations

My diagnosis was that Emily demonstrated speech and language characteristics consistent with an expressive-only SLI. It appeared that her language development course had been fairly normal; thus, differences were not detected until the point in development when children are beginning to add inflectional morphemes to their expressive repertoires. However, it appeared obvious that the child, who was minimally stimulable for production of the grammatical morphemes she omitted, would probably not figure this out on her own without some direct intervention. Given the child's age, too, with formalized literacy learning on the horizon, it was likely that learning to read might be negatively affected by this child's poor expressive language performance. Intervention was strongly recommended.

Step 4: Intervention

- Emily's school administration was reluctant to provide speech treatment services for Emily because her receptive language skills had tested as high as they had. It took a concerted effort by the mother, the school clinician, the classroom teacher, and this clinician to present the rationale for services in such a way that the administration was convinced that this was the appropriate course of action. Emily was scheduled for therapy twice weekly, once in an individual session and the second time in a group with two other children who were working on similar goals.

- Once she began treatment, Emily's mother was counseled about ways to help carry over what Emily learned in her therapy at school into the home environment.

- Emily's best friend Doris, who had assisted with language sample collection, was trained in being a peer tutor for her friend, providing gentle cues to focus Emily's attention when the child omitted a grammatical morpheme that had been targeted in therapy.

Step 5: Outcomes of Intervention

- Emily demonstrated almost immediately that she knew what was expected of her and she paid careful attention to the clinician during her sessions. However, without the clinician's direct model, production of the inflectional morphemes targeted, for example, present progressive, regular past, and plurals, were only rarely observed in therapy, at home, or in the classroom.

- Given the difficulty Emily was having with her goals, the clinician decided to teach Emily orthographic cues that would help provide additional stimulus support for the child's production, that is, instead of hearing the clinician's model, the clinician can hold up a card with a written cue to prompt Emily.

- The clinician is currently investigating the possibility of using a computerized program to assist Emily in hearing, seeing, and remembering when and where the markers need to be included as well as giving her an additional low-risk practice arena outside of the classroom or home environment.

SECTION

4

FORMS FOR EVALUATING PRESCHOOLERS' LANGUAGE AND THEIR SUCCESS IN TREATMENT

T he five forms that follow can be adapted to suit the needs of the clinician and the particular client for whom they will be used. For example, look at the "Form for On-Line Sample Collection." There is a series of eight columns to the right of the space provided for transcribing the utterances produced by the client, clinician, and other conversation partners. These columns can be used to delineate:

1. Speaker?: (CH) Child, (P) Parent, (CL) Clinician, (O) Other

2. Assertive Conversation Act (AA)?

3. Responsive Conversation Act (RA)?

4. Topic Initiation?

5. Topic Maintenance?

6. Topic Tangential?

7. Imitation of Prior Speaker?

8. MLU

They can also be used to identify the eight structures/points earned for Developmental Sentence Scoring in each of the utterances produced by the client or other conversant. You could add an additional column to indicate whether a sentence point had been earned.

Be creative! All children's strengths and needs will be somewhat different so use the forms as a starting point and make changes and additions where it makes sense for the children with language disorders with whom you work.

Form 4–1. Informal Preschool Language Assessment Checklist

(Use in Conjunction with Language Sample Collection)

Examples Observed During Evaluation

PRAGMATICS

    a. Communicative intentions (e.g., requests, demands)

    b. Presupposition (i.e., accommodations to the child's listener)

    c. Conversational discourse rules (e.g., topic initiation, topic maintenance)

SEMANTICS

    a. Vocabulary size (receptive/expressive), as per caregiver's estimate; clinician's estimate

    b. Lexical diversity (type/token ratio)

    c. Semantic relations (e.g., use of agent, location, action, object roles, etc., in combination)

SYNTAX

    a. Sentence types: declaratives
                                 interrogatives
                                 imperatives

    b. Complete versus incomplete sentences, that is, sentence fragments

MORPHOLOGY

    a. Brown's 14 Grammatical Morphemes: Circle presence in obligatory contexts. Note consistency: Never (N), Sometimes (S), Always (A) -ing, in/on, plurals, regular past, irregular past, articles, regular third-person verbs, irregular third-person verbs, uncontractible/ contractible copulas, uncontractible/contractible auxiliaries

    b. Mean Length of Utterance (MLU) estimate:

    c. Corresponding MLU Stage:

    d. Age-Appropriate MLU range for chronological age:

PHONOLOGY

    a. Circle one: Is the child intelligible in connected speech: All of the time? Some of the time? Only if the context is known? Rarely, even if the context is known?

    b. Note individual sound errors observed:

       Note sound patterns observed:

Form 4–2. Form for Language Sample Collection at Home or in the Classroom

What you heard the child say (Try not to add words.)	Context Notes: What was happening at the time?	Interpretation: What do you believe the child meant?

Form 4–3. Form for On-Line Sample Collection

Child's Name: _____

Date of Birth: _____ Age at Testing: _____

Reason For Referral: _____

Date of Sample Collection: _____

Examiner: _____

Form 4–4. Formal Preschool Language Assessment/Evaluation Checklist

Client's Name _____   Date(s) of Testing _____

Date of Birth _____   Personnel Involved _____

Referred by _____   Presenting Concern(s) _____

_____ **Hearing Testing Completed**

    Testing Completed by _____

    Type of Testing Completed _____

    Results _____

    Recommendations _____

    Additional Observations _____

_____ **Cognitive Testing Completed**

    Testing Completed by _____

    Test(s) Completed _____

    Results _____

    Recommendations _____

    Additional Observations _____

_____ **Receptive Language Testing Completed**

    Testing Completed by _____

    Test(s) Completed _____

    Results _____

    Recommendations _____

    Additional Observations _____

_____ **Expressive Language Testing Completed**

    Testing Completed by _____

    Test(s) Completed _____

    Results _____

    Recommendations _____

    Additional Observations _____

_____ **Delineation of Client's Language Strengths**

_____ **Delineation of Client's Language Needs**

Form 4–5. Language Treatment Planning Protocol

Child's Name: _____

Diagnosis: _____

Child's Date of Birth: _____   Date of Evaluation: _____

Child's Age: _____   Place of Evaluation: _____

Examiner(s): _____

Family Members: _____

Summary of Evaluation Results

Standardized Tests Administered and Results

Nonstandardized Probes Administered and Results

Observation of Child's Strengths and Needs

Dynamic Assessment Outcomes

Stimuli:

Reinforcers/Feedback:

Successful Strategies:

Goals/Activities Delineated for Partners in the Treatment Plan

Family/Caregivers: _____

_____

School Personnel: _____

_____

Others: _____

_____

Date/Time/Place of Initial Treatment Session: _____

Initial Treatment Mode Selected: (e.g., Drill, Drill Play, Structured Play, Play) _____

Initial Facilitation Technique to Be Used: (e.g., Modeling, Incidental Teaching, Imitation, Focused Stimulation, Fill-ins)

_____

Initial Selected Activities: _____

_____

Plan for Evaluation of Progress:

SECTION

GLOSSARY

● ●

T his is a glossary of selected terms used in this resource guide. It by no means represents an exhaustive listing of all of the terms one comes across while working in this area.

Assertiveness: a term used by Fey (1986) to describe a co-conversationalist's ability and/or willingness to produce unsolicited **conversational bids** such as statements, requests, and comments. Assertiveness represents one of the two continua that describes young children's use of language.

Assessment: a term used by some clinicians interchangeably with the term *evaluation*. For others, assessment refers to preliminary data collection, perhaps through observation, to determine that a communication problem is present and that a child requires the closer scrutiny of an evaluation.

Bootstrapping: a term used in language acquisition to describe a child's utilization of something already learned to help speculate or guess about some novel linguistic structure or form; for example, children superimpose the very common subject-verb-object structure on passive sentence constructions (a very uncommon structure) to decode them.

Cognition: intellectual capacity, organization, and manipulation that reflects our knowledge of the world and how it works.

Communicative competence: our underlying understanding of the rule system that governs how the communication system operates and our finessing of that system.

Communicative intents: a portion of pragmatics that represents the goals for which language can be used such as requesting, demanding, and labeling.

Conjoining: the production of two or more forms or structures, for example, phrases, clauses, usually with the aid of a part of speech called a conjunction such as *but, if,* and *and*. The period of acquisition during which the child begins conjoining is reflected in one of Brown's Stages of Development (Brown, 1973).

Contrastive analysis: a comparison of two structures or contexts to systematically look for similarities and differences; often used in teaching children to code switch between two different dialects of the same language.

Conversational bids: the taking of a turn within a conversational framework, most often to be assertive (an unsolicited bid) or responsive (a solicited bid).

Dialect: a systematically derived, rule-governed variant of a language with some minor differences in lexical items, grammatical rules, pragmatic conventions, or some combination of these; nonstandard dialects are typically far more like the standard than they are different.

Embedding: the production of sentences with one or more phrases (non NP + VP) and/or clauses (NP + VP) where one clause is designated as the main clause and the remaining clauses and phrases are subordinate or subsumed by the main clause. This represents one major qualitative step in Brown's Stages of Development (Brown, 1973).

Evaluation: For some clinicians this term can be used interchangeably with the term *assessment*. For others, it denotes a comprehensive attempt to establish a diagnosis and determine the scope of a communication problem and follows a preliminary assessment, probably using observation and other less standard methods of data collection.

Fast mapping: one approach to describing children's concept learning where the child uses his first exposure to a word, drawing on the context of that exposure, to speculate about that word's meaning.

Functionalist: the description of someone who views the area of pragmatics as primary in terms of the motivation for language learning; pragmatics represents the essential underpinning for language learning.

Hyperlexia: a phenomenon whereby children normally thought to be too young to read, appear to be reading. In fact, they are probably not engaged in any meaningful symbol decoding, although they are obviously making some connection between the written symbol and the sound it represents. This often is an observed characteristic of children diagnosed with autism spectrum disorder.

Idiolect: an idiosyncratic, minimally communicative attempt at creating a private language that has been observed in the communication of twins and other sibling groups. A rare occurrence, it frequently cannot be understood by anyone outside of the small group of its developers.

Language: a systematic, rule-governed symbol system used for the purposes of communication that represents a socially shared set of conventions for deriving forms and structures. All languages contain aspects of semantics, syntax/morphology, phonology, and pragmatics.

Language difference: the presence of lexical, morphological, syntatic, phonological, and/or pragmatic alternatives to a standard language that are systematic and rule-governed. Dialect differences, such as those few morphological differences that can exist between the language systems of speakers of African American English and Standard English, do not represent disordered or "broken" English but a viable, although somewhat different, language system.

Language disorder: the presence of a language system that is either developing in a manner that is significantly delayed when compared with normal rates of acquisition or the pattern of the development is atypical of normally developing children. Language disorders can manifest themselves across all modalities of language decoding and encoding and may be evident in some or all of the component parts of the communication system, for example, pragmatics, semantics, and syntax.

Language-learning style: a term used to describe the individual differences in language acquisition patterns that are not indicative of pathological deviations from normal development but instead may be different pathways to reaching language competence.

"Late talkers": a term used to describe young preschoolers who are significantly delayed in acquisition of their first vocabulary words and in their combination into two-word utterances. A sizable proportion of these children have been shown to continue to experience language difficulties through age 3 and are diagnosed as SLI.

Mapping: a term used in language development to describe the connection of language symbols with nonlinguistic context. One of the reasons for context-based intervention is to make the child's job of mapping what is being said with the context more obvious and thus an easier task.

Modalities: the forms of manner of language reception or expression available to the child for the purpose of language decoding and encoding, for example, auditory (speech), visual (reading, signed symbols), motor (speech and gestures or signed systems).

Morphemes: the smallest units of meaning in a language. They can be further designated as free (capable of standing alone, e.g., single words) versus bound (they must be connected with another morpheme, e.g., plural marker), inflectional (that appear as suffixes and allow the speaker to be more specific, e.g., plurals, past tense marker) versus derivational (that change words from one class to another, e.g., sad to sadness).

Morphology: the area of language that deals with the acquisition of morphological markers and often with the internal word changes that occur when grammatical changes occur, for example, plurals.

Narratives: a text form that requires the producer to tell a story in a form prescribed by a set of rules referred to as **story grammar**. Narratives can be conveyed in oral or written form.

Pervasive Developmental Disorder (PDD): a controversial label that has been used by some professionals to designate children who manifest atypical behaviors and poor or no communication skills. Often these children have some or many of the characteristics of autism or autism spectrum disorder, but this diagnosis has not been made. As a result the children may not be eligible for potentially helpful services. Some believe that the label of PDD is used when a professional is unsure how to diagnose a child; its use does not provide helpful directions for therapeutic intervention because it is not necessarily accurate or descriptive.

Phonology: the area of language that deals with the acquisition of the sound system of a language including a phoneme inventory, and the rules for combining these phonemes.

Pragmatics: the area of language that focuses on how language is used in different social contexts; Roth and Spekman (1984a) divide pragmatics into the three major portions of communicative intents, presupposition, and discourse.

Presupposition: a portion of pragmatics that refers to the assumptions made about what the listener knows and does not know that guides us in our choices of communicative style to enhance the success of communication with others.

Probes: lists of examples of a particular target or goal that can be used to evaluate whether or not a client has learned the items specifically trained (use probe lists comprised of examples used in therapy) or generalized to similar but untaught examples (probe lists should contain items not specifically taught).

Protodeclaratives: usually emerge prior to the child's production of first real words. They often consist of pointing or showing some object and are used for the purpose of getting an adult's attention.

Protoimperatives: usually emerge prior to the child's production of first real words. They often consist of giving gestures with the intention of getting an adult to help get an object the child cannot get without assistance.

Real word use: a child is credited with using a real word if these three criteria are met: (1) the word attempt must resemble a real word in the language the child is learning, (2) the child's productions must be phonetically consistent, and (3) the child's productions have to be contextually consistent as well.

Responsiveness: one of the two continua (the other being assertiveness) discussed by Fey (1986) that relates to a child's understanding of the basic role of participation in communication. Responsiveness refers to the child's propensity for providing responses to the requests made by a co-conversationalist.

Semantics: the area of language focused on vocabulary development and the development of word combinations to describe the variety of relationships between people, things, and events in the child's world.

Speech acts: these are units of intentionally communicated messages that include not only the speaker's communicative intention but also the listener's ability to interpret the message.

Story grammar: sets of culture-based rules that govern how stories must be constructed to enhance their comprehension by persons in that culture. Stein and Glenn (1979) described a story grammar that specified episode structure.

Syntax: the area of language that focuses on the development of noun phrases and verb phrases into a variety of different grammatical sentence types, for example, declaratives and interrogatives.

Text: a general term that can be used to refer to the production of sets of sentences in stories or in expository form, to name two possibilities. To master text forms, children need to learn something about cohesion, the linguistic devices that help to hold text together in an understandable format such as the use of pronouns with specified referents.

SECTION

INTERNET RESOURCES

SELECTED INTERNET SITES

A number of Internet Web sites provide speech-language pathologists (audiologists and other professionals) with informational resources to enhance their own knowledge base as well as provide their clients and clients' families a continuous updating of information. The following Web sites may be particularly useful to the practitioner who is working with preschool-age children with language disorders or those who have been diagnosed with SLI. Please note that, with the massive proliferation of Web sites, it is virtually impossible to keep entirely up-to-date with what is available to the public on the Internet. So, I am sure that there are many important and useful Web sites that have been omitted. This list is meant to give the reader a place to start.

Internet Sites Developed for Nongovernmental Organizations

http://www.asha.org/
Most members of the American Speech-Language-Hearing Association are aware that their organization has a prodigious Web site that is frequently updated with important information for professionals, students, and consumers. Included are links to professional and consumer information that may be the most useful for our readers. For example, see the following Web site.

http://www.asha.org/consumers/brochures/brochures.htm

This site lists brochures, information packets, booklets, and fact sheets to educate people about services and various speech, language, and hearing disabilities, some of which can be accessed on line. Examples of brochures and information packets are available. Included are questions and answers about child language, child speech and language disorders, and recognizing communication disorders. This site is useful for anyone needing basic information regarding speech, language, and hearing disabilities, for example, parents, classroom teachers, SLPs, and other professionals working with young children.

http://www.hanen.org/

This site describes in detail the Hanen program for speech-language pathologists, parents of children with language delay, and early childhood educators and teachers. There is a link to a resource list for both parents and professionals.

http://www.autism.org/

This is the home page for the Center for the Study of Autism, whose purpose is to provide information to both professionals and parents regarding autism and autism spectrum disorders. The center also sponsors treatment efficacy research. A table of contents guides users through a selection of well-written articles covering common topics of interest including disorder subgroupings, terminology associated with autism and its treatment, related disorders, diagnostic issues, and intervention programming choices.

http://www.dec-sped.org/

The home page of the Division of Early Childhood of the Council for Exceptional Children provides connection to current issues of their publications *Young Exceptional Children* and the *Journal of Early Intervention* as well as the organization's position statements and policies.

http://www.naeyc.org/

This is the home page of the National Association for the Education of Young Children. Four major avenues of information linkages are provided: (1) catalog, with a list of resources available from the organization; (2) children's champion, providing linkages to current, pertinent activity by the United States Congress, research reports, and "Violence prevention tools"; (3) accreditation requirements, for providing day care/preschool programs; and (4) annual conference information.

http://www.childrensdefense.org/

This is the home page of the Children's Defense Fund, which refers to itself as "America's Strongest Voice for All Children." Their motto, prominently displayed on the home page is: "Leave no child behind." Users can link to Current Features, What's New?, Special Reports, Take Action, and Publications. A Parent Resource Network and a Listserv are also available from the home page.

http://www.nbcdi.org/

This is the home page for the National Black Child Development Institute, an organization dedicated to the improvement and protection of the quality of life of African-American children and their families. Users can connect to information regarding the Institute's affiliate network, resource center, publications, and public policy statement.

Internet Sites Developed for Governmental Organizations

http://www.ed.gov/

The home page of the United States Department of Education serves as an entry point for accessing information for professionals and consumers regarding departmental priorities, programs and services provided, and publications and products offered, among other topics. Current updates of administration initiatives and reports are also provided. A list of "most requested items" allows for quick access to a number of topics among them, "Helping Your Child," a valuable set of suggestions for parents. Topics include: "Helping Your Child Get Ready for School" and "Helping Your Child Succeed in School." At least three of these are available in Spanish as well as in English.

http://www.accesseric.org/

This is the home page of the Educational Resources Information Center (ERIC), a national information system established in 1966 for the purpose of providing users with ready access to education-related documents, research reports, and other literature. The Clearinghouse on Elementary and Early Childhood Education, located at the University of Illinois–Champaign-Urbana, allows for easy searches of the ERIC database and the Web site itself, a set of resources for parents (National Parent Information Network), papers prepared for special topics, and a question-answer Internet-based service, as well as a Listserv. The latter provides a forum for discussion of educational topics covering early childhood through middle-level education.

http://www.ed.gov/databases/ERIC_Digests

The ERIC Digests can also be accessed through this site. Updated quarterly, the ERIC Digests are abstracts and summaries of educational topics primarily useful for teachers, administrators, and policy makers, according to the site's text. All records contained in the ERIC Digests contain sufficient identifying information so that the full text can be accessed.

http://www.nectas.unc.edu/

This is the home page of the National Childhood Technical Assistance System. The NECTAS consortium consists of six organizations coordinated through the Frank Porter Graham Child Development Center at the University of North Carolina at Chapel Hill and funded through the United States Office of Special Education Programs (OSEP). From the home page, professionals can: (a) obtain information about governmental policy (e.g., inclusion, the IDEA); (b) find reports on NECTAS activities that have focused on early literacy, developmental delay, among others; (c) find information about OSEP-funded projects; and (d) link to currently available NECTAS publications. Their "Links to Other Resources" is especially helpful in moving through the maze of related government agencies and the information available therein.

http://www2.acf.dhhs.gov/programs/hsb/index.htm

This is the home page for the Head Start program, supported by the Administration for Children and Families of the United States Department of Health and Human Services. The site serves as a resource to persons involved in the provision of Head Start services, parents, and others interested in provision of child development services to children from low-income households. From this site, you can glean information concerning legislative regulations and policies governing Head Start programs, as well as summaries of research findings and statistics for Head Start projects nationwide.

http://www.nmchc.org/

The National Maternal and Child Health Clearinghouse is the home page for the Health Resources and Services Administration, Maternal and Child Bureau, which is funded through the United States Department of Health and Human Services. The purpose of the clearinghouse is to allow for easy dissemination of all of the agency's publications from two-page resource sheets of state-by-state services to complete publications aimed at both professionals and families. Materials related to sudden infant death syndrome receive special focus on this organization's home page.

Additional Web Sites

http://www.kidsource.com/

Although this site is focused on all areas of children's development, there are a number of linkages to information about communication. Specifically, the site can link the reader to articles in ASHA publications regarding children and communication in general. Included in this site is information regarding tips for pragmatic language learning, predicting poor readers, and early identification of speech and language delays and disorders. This site can be a very useful one for parents, teachers, and SLPs wanting some very basic information about language learning as well as other areas of child development. In fact, the home page is set up in such a way that information can be easily delineated for newborns, toddlers, preschoolers, and school-age children (grades K through 12). Note that the topics covered on this site change periodically.

http://www.blankees.com/baby/speech/index.htm

This site provides the reader with lists of developmental milestones for speech and language development from birth to approximately 5 years of age. Warning signs that development is not proceeding normally are also included. This information is presented at a basic level and is useful for parents, teachers, SLPs, and other professionals.

http://www.mankato.msus.edu/dept/comdis/kuster2/sldisorders/childlang.html

This site was developed by Professor Judith Kuster at Mankato State University in Minnesota, and this address allows the user to link to other child language disorder sites. Included in the selection of sites are those that contain questions and answers about child language development and disorders, research in child language disorders, suggestions for intervention for children with pragmatic and/or semantic disorders, language-based learning disabilities, and dyslexia. This site would probably be useful for families and special educators as well as SLPs.

http://members.tripod.com/Caroline_Bowen/home.html

This site is a source for information about a number of topics concerning speech and language but includes a focus on normal language development, Brown's stages, and activities for word-retrieval problems. This site also provides links to other related language sites.

http://www.sd01.k12.id.us/schools/whitney/teachers/clousw/language.htm

This site provides basic definitions for frequently used language terms such as semantics, syntax-morphology, and pragmatics. There is also some information regarding literacy learning and its interface with speech and language development. From here, one can link to the site's author's literacy page that deals with "how-tos" for reading to a child to encourage language growth. Note that this material is presented at a beginning level and is directed at parents but may be useful for teachers and SLPs as well.

REFERENCES

Achenbach, T. (1991). *Manual for the Child Behavior Checklist/4–18 and 1991 Profile*. Burlington, VT: University of Vermont Department of Psychiatry.

Applebee, A. (1978). *The child's concept of story*. Chicago: The University of Chicago Press.

ASHA Technical Report. (1988). *Issues in determining eligibility for language intervention*. ASHA Desk Reference, Volume III (pp. 207–215). Rockville, MD: American Speech-Language-Hearing Association.

ASHA 1997 Omnibus Survey. *ASHA science and research*. Rockville, MD: American Speech-Language-Hearing Association.

American Speech-Language-Hearing Association. (1983). Social dialects: A position paper. *Asha, 25*(1), 23–24.

ASHA Committee on Language. (1983). Definition of language. *Asha, 25* (6), 44.

Bain, B., & Dollaghan, C. (1991). The notion of clinically significant change. *Language, Speech and Hearing Services in Schools, 22*, 264–270.

Bain, B., & Olswang, L. (1995). Examining readiness for learning two-word utterances by children with specific expressive language impairment: Dynamic assessment validation. *American Journal of Speech-Language Pathology, 4*(1), 81–92.

Bandura, A., & Harris, M. (1966). Modifications of syntactic style. *Journal of Experimental Child Psychology, 4*, 341–352.

Bates, E. (1976). *Language and context: Studies in the acquisition of pragmatics*. New York: Academic Press.

Bates, E., & MacWhinney, B. (1982). Functionalist approaches to grammar. In E. Warner & L. Gleitman (Eds.), *Language acquisition: The state of the art* (pp. 173–218). New York: Cambridge University Press.

Bedrosian, J. (1985). An approach to developing conversational competence. In D. Ripich & F. Spinelli (Eds.), *School discourse problems* (pp. 231–255). San Diego: College-Hill Press.

Beitchman, J. (1985). Speech and language impairment and psychiatric risk: Toward a model of neurodevelopmental immaturity. *Psychiatric Clinics of North America, 8*, 721–735.

Beitchman, J., Wilson, B., Brownlie, E., Walters, H., & Lancee, W. (1996). Long-term consistency in speech/language profiles: I. Developmental and academic outcomes. *Journal of the American Academy of Child and Adolescent Psychiatry, 35*, 804–814.

Benedict, H. (1979). Early lexical developer: Comprehension and production. *Journal of Child Language, 6,* 183–200.

Bishop, D. (1979). Comprehension in development language disorders. *Developmental Medicine and Child Neurology 21,* 225–238.

Bishop, D., & Edmundson, A. (1987). Specific language impairment as a maturational lag: Evidence from longitudinal data on language and motor development. *Developmental Medicine and Child Neurology, 29,* 442–459.

Bloom, L. (1970). *Language development: Form and function of emerging grammars.* Cambridge: MIT Press.

Bloom, L. (1973). *One word at a time: The use of single-word utterances before syntax.* The Hague: Mouton.

Bloom, L., & Lahey, M. (1978). *Language development and language disorders.* New York: Wiley.

Brinton, B., & Fujiki, M. (1989). *Conversational management with language-impaired children: Pragmatic assessment and intervention.* Rockville, MD: Aspen Publishers.

Brinton, B., & Fujiki, M. (1995). Conversational intervention with children with language impairment. In M. Fey, J. Windsor, & S. Warren (Eds.), *Language intervention: Preschool through the primary school years* (pp. 183–212). Baltimore: Paul H. Brookes Publishing Co.

Brown, J., Redmond, A., Bass, K., Liebergott, J., & Swope, S. (1975). *Symbolic play in normal and language-impaired children.* Paper presented at the Annual Convention of the American Speech-Language-Hearing Association, Washington, DC.

Brown, L., Sherbenou, R., & Johnson, S. (1982). *Test of nonverbal intelligence.* Austin, TX: Pro-Ed.

Brown, R. (1973). *A first language: The early stages.* Cambridge: Harvard University Press.

Burgemeister, B., Blum, H., & Lorge, I. (1972). *The Columbia Mental Maturity Scale.* New York: Psychological Corporation.

Camarata, S., & Nelson, K. (1992). Treatment efficiency as a function of target selection in the remediation of child language disorders. *Clinical Linguistics and Phonetics, 6,* 167–178.

Camarata, S., Nelson, K., & Camarata, M. (1994). Comparison of conversational recasting and imitative procedures for training grammatical structures in children with specific language impairment. *Journal of Speech and Hearing Research, 37,* 1414–1423.

Campbell, T., & Bain, B. (1991). How long to treat: A multiple outcome approach. *Language, Speech, and Hearing Services in Schools, 22,* 271–276.

Campbell, T., & Shriberg, L. (1982). Association among pragmatic functions, linguistic stress, and natural phonological processes in speech-delayed children. *Journal of Speech and Hearing Research, 25,* 547–553.

Carrow-Woolfolk, E. (1999). *Test for auditory comprehension of language* (3rd ed.). Austin, TX: Pro-Ed.

Catts, H., & Kamhi, A. (Eds.) (1998). *Language and reading disabilities.* Boston: Allyn & Bacon.

Chapman, R. (1978). Comprehension strategies in children. In J. Kavanaugh & W. Strange (Eds.), *Speech and language in the laboratory, school and clinic.* Cambridge: MIT Press.

Coggins, T., & Carpenter, R. (1981). The communicative intention inventory. *Journal of Applied Psycholinguistics, 2,* 213–234.

Conti-Ramsden, G., Crutchley, A., & Botting, N. (1997). The extent to which psychometric tests differentiate subgroups of children with SLI. *Journal of Speech and Hearing Research, 40,* 765–777.

Courtwright, J., & Courtwright, I. (1976). Imitative modeling as a theoretical base for instructing language disordered children. *Journal of Speech and Hearing Research, 19,* 655–663.

Craig, H., & Washington, J. (1993). The access behaviors of children with specific language impairment. *Journal of Speech and Hearing Research, 36,* 322–337.

Craig, H., & Washington, J. (1994). The complex syntax skills of poor, urban, African-American preschoolers at school entry. *Language, Speech and Hearing Services in Schools, 25,* 181–190.

Crary, M. (1993). *Developmental motor speech disorders.* San Diego: Singular Publishing Group.

Crystal, D. (1982). *Profiling linguistic disability.* London, UK: Edward Arnold.

Crystal, D., Fletcher, P., & Garman, M. (1989). *The grammatical analysis of language disability.* New York: Elsevier.

de Villiers, J., Roeper, T., & de Villiers, P. (1999, November). *What every five-year-old should know: Syntax, semantics and pragmatics.* A seminar presented to the annual convention of the American Speech-Language-Hearing Association, San Francisco.

Dunn, L., & Dunn, L. (1997). *Peabody Picture Vocabulary Test* (3rd ed.). Circle Pines, MN: American Guidance Service.

Dunst, C., Trivette, C., & Deal, A. (1988). *Enabling and empowering families: Principles and guidelines for practice.* Cambridge, MA: Brookline Books.

Ellis Weismer, S., & Murray-Branch, J. (1989). Modeling versus modeling plus evoked production training: A comparison of two language intervention methods. *Journal of Speech and Hearing Disorders, 54,* 269–281.

Fenson, L., Dale, P., Reznick, S., Thal, D., Bates, E., Hartung, J., Pethick, S., & Reilly, J. (1993). *The MacArthur Communicative Development Inventories.* San Diego: Singular Publishing.

Fewell, R., Snyder, P., Sexton, D., Bertrand, S., & Hookless, M. (1991). Implementing IFSPs in Louisiana: Different formats for family-centered practices under Part II. *Topics in Early Childhood Special Education II,* 54–65.

Fey, M. (1986). *Language intervention with young children.* Needham Heights, MA: Allyn & Bacon.

Fey, M. (1988). Dismissal criteria for the language-impaired child. In D. Yoder & R. Kent (Eds.), *Decision making in speech-language pathology* (pp. 50–54). Toronto: B. C. Decker.

Fey, M., & Cleave, P. (1990). Early language intervention. *Seminars in Speech and Language, 11,* 165–181.

Fey, M., Cleave, P., Long, S., & Hughes, D. (1993). Two approaches to the facilitation of grammar in children with language impairment: An experimental evaluation. *Journal of Speech and Hearing Research, 36,* 141–157.

Fey, M., Leonard, L., Fey, S., & O'Connor, K. (1978). *The intent to communicate in language-impaired children.* A paper presented at The Boston University Conference on Language Development, Boston.

Fey, M., Long, S., & Cleave, P. (1994). Reconsideration of IQ criteria in the definition of specific language impairment. In R. Watkins & M. Rice (Eds.), *Specific language impairments in children* (pp. 161–178). Baltimore: Paul H. Brookes Publishing Co.

FIRST STEPS: *Supporting early language development: Trainer's Manual.* Portland, OR: Educational Productions, Inc.

Friedman, P., & Friedman, K. (1980). Accounting for individual differences when comparing the effectiveness of remedial language teaching methods. *Applied Psycholinguistics, 1,* 151–170.

Gallagher, T. (1983). Preassessment: A procedure for accommodating language variability. In T. Gallagher & C. Prutting (Eds.), *Pragmatic assessment and intervention: Issues in language* (pp. 1–28). San Diego: College-Hill Press.

Gallagher, T., & Darnton, B. (1978). Conversational aspects of the speech of language disordered children: Revision behaviors. *Journal of Speech and Hearing Research, 21,* 118–135.

Gillon, G. (2000). The efficacy of phonological awareness intervention for children with spoken language impairment. *Language, Speech, and Hearing Services in Schools, 31,* 126–147.

Giralometto, L., Greenberg, J., & Manolson, H. (1986). *Developing dialogue skills: The Hanen early language parent program.* New York: Thieme Medical Publishers.

Goldstein, B. (2000). *Cultural and linguistic diversity resource guide for speech-language pathologists.* San Diego: Singular/Thomson Learning.

Gopnik, M., & Crago, M. (1991). Familial aggregation of a developmental language disorder. *Cognition, 39,* 1–50.

Gottsleben, R., Tyack, D., & Buschini, G. (1974). Three case studies in language training: Applied linguistics. *Journal of Speech and Hearing Disorders, 39,* 213–241.

Grunwell, P. (1987). *Clinical phonology* (2nd ed.). Baltimore, MD: Williams & Wilkins.

Grunwell, P. (1992). Assessment of child phonology in the clinical context. In C. Ferguson, L. Menn, & C. Stoel-Gammon (Eds.), *Phonological development: Models, research implications* (pp. 457–483). Timonium, MD: York Press.

Guralnick, M, (1997). *The effectiveness of early intervention.* Baltimore: Paul H. Brookes.

Hall, P. (1999). The oral mechanism (2nd ed.). In J. Tomblin, H. Morris, & D. Spriestersbach (Eds.), *Diagnosis in speech-language pathology* (pp. 91–128). San Diego: Singular Publishing Group.

Hall, P., Jordan, L., & Robin, D. (1993). *Developmental apraxia of speech: Theory and clinical practice.* Austin, TX: Pro-Ed.

Hegde, M., & Gierut, J. (1979). The operant training and generalization of pronouns and a verb form in a language delayed child. *Journal of Communication Disorders, 12*, 23–24.

Hodson, B., & Paden, E. (1991). *Targeting intelligible speech: A phonological approach to remediation* (2nd ed.). Austin, TX: Pro-Ed.

Hresko, W., Reid, D., & Hammill, D. (1999). *Test of Early Language Development–3 (TELD–3)*. Austin, TX: Pro-Ed.

Hughes, D. (1985). *Language treatment and generalization*. San Diego: College-Hill Press.

Hughes, D., McGillivray, L., & Schmidek, M. (1997). *Guide to narrative language: Procedures for assessment*. Eau Claire, WI: Thinking Publications.

Johnston, J., & Ellis Weismer, S. (1983). Mental rotation abilities in language-disordered children. *Journal of Speech and Hearing Research, 26*, 397–403.

Kaufman, A., & Kaufman, N. (1983). *Kaufman Assessment Battery for Children*. Circle Pines, MN: American Guidance Service.

Kelly, E., & Conture, E. (1992). Speaking rates, response time latencies, and interrupting behaviors of young stutterers, non-stutterers, and their mothers. *Journal of Speech and Hearing Research, 35*, 1256–1267.

Kent, R. (1994). *Reference manual for communicative sciences and disorders: Speech and language*. Austin, TX: Pro-Ed.

Leach, E. (1972). Interrogation: A model and some implications. *Journal of Speech and Hearing Disorders, 37*, 33–46.

Leadholm, B., & Miller, J. (1992). *Language sample analysis: The Wisconsin guide*. Madison, WI: Wisconsin Department of Public Instruction.

Lee, L. (1974). *Developmental sentence analysis*. Evanston, IL: Northwestern University Press.

Leonard, L. (1972). What is deviant language? *Journal of Speech and Hearing Disorders, 37*, 427–446.

Leonard, L. (1981). Facilitating language skills in children with specific language impairment: A review. *Applied Psycholinguistics, 2*, 89–118.

Leonard, L. (1998). *Children with specific language impairment*. Cambridge, MA: The MIT Press.

Leonard, L., Eyer, J., Bedore, L., & Grela, B. (1997). Three accounts of the grammatical morpheme difficulties of English speaking children with specific language impairment. *Journal of Speech and Hearing Research, 40*, 741–753.

Leonard, L., & Leonard, J. (1985). The contribution of phonetic context to an unusual phonological pattern: A case study. *Language, Speech, and Hearing Services in Schools, 16*, 110–118.

Leonard, L., McGregor, K., & Allen, G. (1992). Grammatical morphology and speech perception in children with specific language impairment. *Journal of Speech and Hearing Research, 35*, 1076–1085.

Leonard, L., Prutting, C., Perozzi, J., & Berkeley, R. (1978). Nonstandardized approaches to the assessment of language behaviors. *Asha, 20*, 371–379.

Leonard, L., Schwartz, R., Chapman, K., Rowan, L., Prelock, P., Terrell, B., Weiss, A., & Messick, C. (1982). Early lexical acquisition in children with specific language impairment. *Journal of Speech and Hearing Research, 25*, 554–564.

Lidz, C., & Pena, E. (1996). Dynamic assessment: The model, its relevance as a non-biased approach, and its application to Latino American preschool children. *Language, Speech, and Hearing Services in Schools, 27*, 367–372.

Long, S., Fey, M., & Channell, R. (2000). *Computerized profiling* (Version 9.27). Cleveland, OH: Case Western Reserve University.

Lund, N., & Duchan, J. (1993). *Assessing children's language in naturalistic contexts* (3rd ed.). Englewood Cliffs, NJ: Prentice Hall.

Lynch, E., & Hanson, M. (Eds.) (1998). *Developing cross-cultural competencies. A guide for working with young children and their families* (2nd ed.). Baltimore: Paul H. Brookes Publishing Co.

MacDonald, J. (1989). *Becoming partners with children: From play to conversation*. San Antonio, TX: Special Press.

MacDonald, J., & Carroll, J. (1992). A social partnership model for assessing early communication development: An intervention model for preconversational children. *Language, Speech, and Hearing Services in Schools, 23*, 113–124.

MacWhinney, B. (1995). *The CHILDES project: Tools for analyzing talk*. Hillsdale, NJ: Lawrence Erlbaum Associates.

Manolson, A. (1992). *It takes two to talk: A parent's guide to helping children communicate*. Toronto, Ontario: The Hanen Centre.

McCauley, R., & Swisher, L. (1984). Psychometric review of language and articulation tests for preschool children. *Journal of Speech and Hearing Disorders, 49,* 34–42.

Merzenich, M., Jenkins, W., Johnston, P., Schreiner, C., Miller, S., & Tallal, P. (1996). Temporal processing deficits of language learning impaired children ameliorated by training. *Science, 271,* 77–81.

Miller, J. (1981). *Assessing language production in children.* Baltimore: University Park Press.

Miller, J., & Chapman, R. (1981). The relation between age and mean length of utterance in morphemes. *Journal of Speech and Hearing Research, 24,* 154–161.

Miller, J., & Chapman, R. (1993). *SALT: Systematic analysis of language transcripts (computer programs to analyze language samples).* Madison, WI: Language Analysis Laboratory, Wisconsin Center, University of Wisconsin–Madison.

Miller, J., Chapman, R., Branston, M., & Reichle, J. (1980). Language comprehension in sensory motor stages 5 and 6. *Journal of Speech and Hearing Research, 23,* 1–12.

Moorehead, D., & Ingram, D. (1973). The development of base syntax in normal and linguistically deviant children. *Journal of Speech and Hearing Research, 16,* 330–352.

Mulac, A., & Tomlinson, C. (1977). Generalization of an operant remediation program for syntax with language-delayed children. *Journal of Communication Disorders, 10,* 231–244.

National Institute on Deafness and Other Communication Disorders. (1995). *National strategic research plan for language and language impairments, balance, balance disorders, and voice and voice disorders.* (NIH Publication No. 97-3217). Bethesda, MD: Author.

Nelson, K. (1973). Structure and strategy in learning to talk. *Monographs of the Society for Research in Child Development, 38.*

Newcomer, P., & Hammill, D. (1992). *Test of Language Development—Primary 2.* Austin, TX: Pro-Ed.

Newcomer, P., & Hammill, D. (1997). *Test of Language Development—Primary 3.* Austin, TX: Pro-Ed.

Oetting, J., Rice, M., & Swank, L. (1995). Quick incidental learning (QUIL) of words by school-age children with and without SLI. *Journal of Speech and Hearing Research, 38,* 434–445.

Olswang, L., & Bain, B. (1991a). Intervention issues for toddlers with specific language impairments. *Topics in Language Disorders, 11,* 69–86.

Olswang, L., & Bain, B. (1991b). When to recommend intervention. *Language, Speech, and Hearing Services in Schools, 22,* 255–263.

Olswang, L., & Bain, B. (1994). Data collection: Monitoring children's treatment progress. *American Journal of Speech-Language Pathology, 3,* 55–66.

Olswang, L., Bain, B., & Johnson, G. (1992). The zone of proximal development: Dynamic assessment of language disordered children. In S. Warren & J. Reichle (Eds.), *Perspectives on communication and language intervention: Development, assessment, and remediation* (pp. 187–216). Baltimore: Paul H. Brookes, Publishing Co.

Olswang, L., Kriegsman, E., & Mastergeorge, A. (1992). Facilitating functional requesting in pragmatically impaired children. *Language, Speech, and Hearing Services in Schools, 13,* 202–223.

Owens, R. (1999). *Language disorders: A functional approach to assessment and intervention* (3rd ed.). Boston: Allyn & Bacon.

Owens, R. (2001). *Language development: An introduction* (5th ed.). Boston: Allyn & Bacon.

Parnell, M., Patterson, S., & Harding, M. (1984). Answers to Wh-questions: A developmental study. *Journal of Speech and Hearing Research, 27,* 297–305.

Paul, R. (1991). Profiles of toddlers with slow expressive language development. *Topics in Language Disorders, 11*(4), 1–13.

Paul, R. (1995). *Language disorders from infancy through adolescence: Assessment and intervention.* St. Louis: Mosby-Year Book, Inc.

Paul, R., Spangle-Looney, S., & Dahm, P. (1991). Communication and socialization skills at ages 2 and 3 in "late talking" young children. *Journal of Speech and Hearing Disorders, 34,* 858–865.

Paul, R., & Smith, R. (1993). Narrative skills in 4-year-olds with normal, impaired, and late-developing language. *Journal of Speech and Hearing Research, 36,* 592–598.

Paul, R., & Unkefer, C. (November, 1995, as cited in Leonard, 1995). *Familiarity in early language delay.* Poster presented at the annual convention of the American Speech-Language-Hearing Association, Orlando, FL.

Plante, E. (1996). Phenotypic variability in brain-behavior studies of specific language impairment. In M. Rice (Ed.), *Toward a genetics of language* (pp. 317–335). Hillsdale, NJ: Lawrence Erlbaum.

Pletcher, L. (1995). Family-centered practices: A training guide. Raleigh, NC: ARCH National Resource Center for Respite and Crisis Care Services.

Preisser, D., Hodson, B., & Paden, E. (1988). Developmental phonology: 18–29 months. *Journal of Speech and Hearing Disorders, 53,* 125–130.

Prelock, P. (1999). *Serving children with autism spectrum disorders and their families.* Pittsburgh, PA: RTN, Inc.

Prutting, C. (1979). Process: The action of moving forward progressively from one point to another on the way to completion. *Journal of Speech and Hearing Disorders, 44,* 3–30.

Ramey, C., & Ramey, S. (1998). Early intervention and early experiences. *American Psychologist, 53*(2), 109–120.

Rapin, I. (1996). Developmental language disorders: A clinical update. *Journal of Child Psychology and Psychiatry, 37,* 643–655.

Rapin, I., & Allen, D. (1987). Developmental dysphasia and autism in preschool children: Characteristics and subtypes. In *Proceedings of the First International Symposium for Specific Speech and Language Disorders in Children* (pp. 20–35). Brentford, UK: Association for All Speech Impaired Children.

Records, N., & Weiss, A. (1990). Clinical judgement: An overview. *Journal of Childhood Communication Disorders, 13,* 153–165.

Rescorla, L. (1989). The Language Development Survey: A screening tool for delayed language in toddlers. *Journal of Speech and Hearing Disorders, 54,* 587–599.

Rescorla, L., & Bernstein Ratner, N. (1996). Phonetic profiles of toddlers with specific expressive language impairment (SLI-E). *Journal of Speech and Hearing Research, 39,* 153–165.

Rescorla, L., & Goosens, M. (1992). Symbolic play development in toddlers with expressive specific language impairment (SLI-E). *Journal of Speech and Hearing Research, 35,* 1290–1302.

Retherford, K. (1993). *Guide to analysis of language transcripts* (2nd ed.). Eau Claire, WI: Thinking Publications.

Retherford, K., Schwartz, B., & Chapman, R. (1981). Semantic roles in mother and child speech: Who tunes to whom? *Journal of Child Language, 8,* 583–608.

Retherford-Stickler, K. (1996). *NCA: Normal Communication acquisition: An animated database of behaviors* (CD-ROM). Eau Claire, WI: Thinking Publications.

Rice, M. (1993). "Don't talk to him: He's weird": The role of language in early social interactions. In A. Kaiser & D. Gray (Eds.), *Enhancing children's communication: Research foundations for intervention* (pp. 139–158). Baltimore: Paul H. Brookes Publishing Co.

Rice, M. (1994). Grammatical categories of children with specific language impairments. In R. Watkins & M. Rice (Eds.), *Specific language impairments in children* (pp. 69–89). Baltimore: Paul H. Brookes Publishing Co.

Rice, M. (1997). Speaking out: Evaluating new training programs for language impairment. *Asha, 39,* 13.

Rice, M., Buhr, J., & Oetting, J. (1992). Specific language impaired children's quick incidental learning of words: The effect of a pause. *Journal of Speech and Hearing Research, 35,* 1040–1048.

Rice, M., Oetting, J., Marquis, J., Bode, J., & Poe, S. (1994). Frequency of input effects on word comprehension of children with specific language impairment. *Journal of Speech and Hearing Research, 37,* 106–122.

Rice, M., & Wexler, K. (1995). Extended optional infinitive (EOI) account of specific language impairment. In D. MacLaughlin & S. McEwen (Eds.), *Proceedings of the 19th Annual Boston University Conference on Language Development, 2,* (pp. 451–462). Somerville, MA: Cascadilla Press.

Roth, F., & Clark, D. (1987). Symbolic play and social participation abilities of language-impaired and normally-developing children. *Journal of Speech and Hearing Disorders, 52,* 17–29.

Roth, F., & Spekman, N. (1984a). Assessing the pragmatic abilities of children: Part 1. Organizational framework and assessment parameters. *Journal of Speech and Hearing Disorders, 49,* 2–11.

Roth, F., & Spekman, N. (1984b). Assessing the pragmatic abilities of children: Part 2. Guidelines, considerations, and specific evaluation procedures. *Journal of Speech and Hearing Disorders, 49,* 12–17.

Scarborough, H. (1990). Very early language deficits in dyslexic children. *Child Development, 61,* 1228–1243.

Scarborough, H., & Dobrich, W. (1990). Development of children with early language delay. *Journal of Speech and Hearing Research, 33,* 70–83.

Seymour, H. (June, 2000). *The development of a dialect sensitive language test.* An invited presentation to the 21st Symposium on Research in Child Language Disorders, Madison, WI.

Shriberg, L., & Kwiatkowski, J. (1982). Phonological disorders II: A conceptual framework for management. *Journal of Speech and Hearing Research, 47,* 242–255.

Shriberg, L., & Kwiatkowski, J. (1994). Developmental phonological disorders I: A clinical profile. *Journal of Speech and Hearing Research, 37,* 1100–1126.

Smit, A., Hand, L., Freilinger, J., Bernthal, J., & Bird, A. (1990). The Iowa articulation norms project and its Nebraska replication. *Journal of Speech and Hearing Disorders, 55,* 779–798.

Snow, C., Burns, M., & Griffin, P. (Eds.). (1998). *Preventing reading difficulties in young children.* Committee on the Prevention of Reading Difficulties in Young Children. Washington, DC: National Academy Press.

Snyder, L. (1980). Have we prepared the language disordered child for school? *Topics in Language Disorders, 1,* 29–45.

Stark, R., & Tallal, P. (1981). Selection of children with specific language deficits. *Journal of Speech and Hearing Disorders, 46,* 114–122.

Stein, N., & Glenn, C. (1979). An analysis of story comprehension in elementary school children. In R. Freedle (Ed.), *New directions in discourse processing: Vol. 2.* (pp. 53–120). Norwood, NJ: Ablex.

Stoel-Gammon, C., & Dunn, C. (1985). *Normal and disordered phonology in children.* Austin, TX: Pro-Ed.

Tallal, P. (1997). Speaking out: Evaluating new training programs for language impairment. *Asha, 39,* 12.

Tallal, P., Ross, R., & Curtiss, S. (1989). Familial aggregation in specific language impairment. *Journal of Speech and Hearing Disorders, 54,* 167–173.

Templin, M. (1957). *Certain language skills in children.* Minneapolis: University of Minnesota Press.

Thal, D., Bates, E., Goodman, J., & Jahn-Samilo, J. (1997). Continuity of language abilities: An exploratory study of late- and early-talking toddlers. *Developmental Neuropsychology, 13*(3), 239–274.

Thal, D., Tobias, S., & Morrison, D. (1991). Language and gesture in late talkers: A one-year follow-up. *Journal of Speech and Hearing Research, 34,* 604–612.

Tomblin, J. (1989). Familial concentration of developmental language impairment. *Journal of Speech and Hearing Disorders, 54,* 287–295.

Tomblin, J., Ellis Weismer, S., & Weiss, A. (1996). *Questionnaires for classroom teachers, SLPs and parents regarding children's communication competencies.* Unpublished data collection protocols. Child Language Research Center, University of Iowa, Iowa City, IA.

Tomblin, J., Freese, P., & Records, N. (1992). Diagnosing specific language impairment in adults for the purpose of pedigree analysis. *Journal of Speech and Hearing Research, 38,* 832–843.

Tomblin, J., Morris, H., & Spriestersbach, D. (Eds.) (1999). *Diagnosis in speech-language pathology* (2nd ed.). San Diego: Singular Publishing Group, Inc.

Tomblin, J., Records, N., Buckwalter, P., Zhang, X., Smith, E., & O'Brien, M. (1997). Prevalence of specific language impairment in kindergarten children. *Journal of Speech, Language, and Hearing Research, 40,* 1245–1260.

Tomblin, J., Records, N., & Zhang, X. (1996). A system for the diagnosis of specific language impairments in kindergarten children. *Journal of Speech and Hearing Research, 39,* 1284–1294.

Trauner, D., Wulfeck, B., Tallal, P., & Hesselink, J. (1995, as cited in Leonard, 1998). *Neurologic and MRI profiles of language impaired children.* (Tech. Rep. CVD-9513). Center for Research in Language, University of California, San Diego.

Tyack, D., & Gottsleben, R. (1977). *Language sampling, analysis, and training: A handbook for teachers and clinicians.* Palo Alto, CA: Consulting Psychologists Press.

Tyack, D., & Ingram, D. (1977). Children's production and comprehension of questions. *Journal of Child Language, 4,* 211–224.

van Kleeck, A. (1994). Potential cultural bias in training parents as conversational partners with their children who have delays in language development. *American Journal of Speech-Language Pathology, 3,* 67–78.

van Kleeck, A., Gillam, R., & McFadden, T. (1998). A study of classroom-based phonological awareness training for preschoolers with speech and/or language disorders. *American Journal of Speech-Language Pathology, 7,* 65–76.

Vaughn-Cooke, F. (1986). The challenge of assessing the language of non-mainstream speakers. In O. Taylor (Ed.), *Treatment of communicative disorders in culturally and linguistically diverse populations* (pp. 23–48). Boston: College-Hill Press.

Velleman, S., & Strand, K. (1994). Developmental verbal dyspraxia. In J. Bernthal & N. Bankson (Eds.), *Child phonology: Characteristics, assessment, and intervention with special populations* (pp. 110–139). New York: Thieme Medical Publishers.

Warren, S., McQuarter, R., & Rogers-Warren, A. (1984). The effects of mands and models on the speech of unresponsive language-delayed preschool children. *Journal of Speech and Hearing Disorders, 49,* 43–52.

Washington, J., & Craig, H. (1994). Dialectal forms during discourse of poor, urban, African-American preschoolers. *Journal of Speech and Hearing Research, 37,* 819–823.

Watkins, R. (1994). Specific language impairments in children: An introduction (pp. 1–15). In R. Watkins & M. Rice (Eds.), *Specific language impairments in children.* Baltimore: Paul H. Brookes Publishing Co.

Watkins, R., & Rice, M., (Eds.) (1994). *Specific language impairments in children.* Baltimore: Paul H. Brookes Publishing Co.

Watkins, R., Rice, M., & Moltz, C. (1993). Verb use by language impaired and normally developing children. *First Language, 37,* 133–143.

Wechsler Intelligence Scale for Children (Revised 1974). New York: The Psychological Corporation.

Wechsler Preschool and Primary Scale of Intelligence (Revised 1989). New York: The Psychological Corporation.

Weiss, A. (1997). Planning language intervention for young children. In D. Bernstein & E. Tiegerman (Eds.), *Language and communication disorders in children* (3rd ed.). (pp. 272–323). New York: MacMillan Publishing Co.

Weiss, A., & Nakamura, M. (1992). Children with normal language skills in preschool classrooms for children with language impairments: Differences in modeling style. *Language, Speech, and Hearing Services in Schools, 23,* 64–70.

Weiss, A., Tomblin, J., Buckwalter, P., & Zhang, X. (July, 1999). *Demographics of speech sound disorders in a second grade cohort.* A paper presented to the annual Child Phonology Conference, Bangor, Wales.

Weiss, A., Tomblin, J., & Robin, D. (1999). Language disorders. In J. Tomblin, H. Morris, & D. Spriestersbach (Eds.) (2nd ed.), *Diagnosis in speech-language pathology* (pp. 129-173). San Diego: Singular Publishing Group.

Weiss, R. (1981). INREAL intervention for language handicapped and bilingual children. *Journal of the Division of Early Childhood, 4,* 40–51.

Wells, G. (1985). *Language development in the preschool years.* New York: Cambridge University Press.

Westby, C. (1994). The effects of culture on genre, structure, and style of oral and written texts (pp. 180–218). In G. Wallach & K. Butler (Eds.), *Language learning disability in school-age children and adolescents: Some principles and applications.* Boston: Allyn & Bacon.

Whitehurst, G., Fischel, J., Arnold, G., & Lonigan, C. (1992). Evaluating outcomes with children with expressive language delay (pp. 277–313). In S. Warren & J. Reichle (Eds.), *Causes and effects in communication and language intervention.* Baltimore: Paul H. Brookes.

Wilcox, M. J., & Leonard, L. (1978). Experimental acquisition of wh-questions in language-disordered children. *Journal of Speech and Hearing Research, 21,* 220–239.

Wolfram, W. (1991). *Dialects and American English.* Englewood Cliffs, NJ: Prentice Hall.

Wyatt, T. (1997). Assessment issues with multicultural populations (pp. 379–425). In D. Battle (Ed.). (2nd ed.), *Communication disorders in multicultural populations.* Boston: Butterworth-Heinemann.

Yoder, P., Kaiser, A., & Alpert, C. (1991). An exploratory study of the interaction between language teaching methods and child characteristics. *Journal of Speech and Hearing Research, 34,* 155–167.

Zimmerman, I., Steiner, V., & Pond, R. (1992). *Preschool Language Scale-3.* San Antonio, TX: The Psychological Corporation.

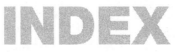

●●

B

Brown's 14 Grammatical Morphemes, 88–89, 145

C

Case history taking
  legal issues, 45
  preassessment, 31, 45–47
Case studies/clinical examples
  facilitation intervention, 107
  late talker, 144–146
  SLI (specific language impairment), 147–148
CHAT (Codes for the Human Analysis of Transcripts), 93
Checklists. See Forms
Child Behavior Checklist (CBCL), 52
CHILDES (Child Language Data Exchange System), 93–94
Children's Defense Fund Web site, 162
CLAN (Computerized Language Analysis), 93
Clinical examples/case studies
  facilitation intervention, 107
  late talker, 144–146
  SLI (specific language impairment), 147–148
Codes for the Human Analysis of Transcripts (CHAT). See CHAT
Codeswitching, 4
Columbia Mental Maturity Scale (CMMS), 51
Comprehension. See also Syntax
  deficits, 23
Computerized Language Analysis (CLAN). See CLAN (Computerized Language Analysis)
Conversation
  assertive partners, 9, 82
  partners, 81–82
  "passive," 145
  recasting/expatiation, 123–124, 135
CP (Computerized Profiling), 94–95
Curricular Competencies Checklist, 37–38

D

Day care placement, 116–117
Development. See Language development
Developmental milestone Web site, 164
Dialect
  ASHA Position Paper on Dialects, 3
  Ebonics, 3–4
DSS (developmental sentence scoring), 147, 148
  language samples, 80, 89–90, 93
Dyspraxia, verbal, 16

E

Ebonics, 3–4
ECO Program intervention, 112
Elicitation techniques, language samples, 83

ERIC (Educational Resources Information Center) Internet sites, 163
Etiology, 18–22
Evaluation. See Assessment
Expressive language, 18, 23, 56, 66–69

F

Family
  disorder clusters, 12
  IFSP (individualized family service plan), 104
  (Family, continued)
  intervention, 102, 103
    carryover, 146, 148
    compliance, 105
    ECO Program intervention, 112
    efficacy, 134
    family-centered, 109–111, 112, 113
    First Steps: Supporting Early Language Development, 113
    Hanen Approach intervention, 112
  and language development, 12
  and language sample collection, 81–82, 103
  preassessment information collection, 42–44
FastForward training program, 19
First Steps: Supporting Early Language Development, 113
Formal Preschool Language Assesment/Evaluation Checklist, 154
Forms. See also Test instruments
  Curricular Competencies Checklist, 37–38
  Discourse Skills Checklist: A Molar Analysis, 31, 32–33
  Formal Preschool Language Assesment/Evaluation Checklist, 154
  Informal Preschool Language Assessment Checklist, 151
  intervention measures, 150–155
    overview, 150
  Language Sample Collection
    classroom/home, 152
    on-line, 153
  Language Treatment Planning Protocol, 155
  Preassessment Questionnaire, 34–36
  Speech-Language Service Delivery Checklist, 39–40

G

Genetics, 12, 21, 48
Goals, language (for 5-year-olds), 99
Governmental organization Internet sites, 162–163

H

Hanen Approach intervention, 112
  Web site, 162
Head Start Web site, 163
History, case, preassessment, 31, 45–47
Hyperlexia, 53